WCC
Exam
SECRETS

Study Guide
Your Key to Exam Success

**WCC Test Review for the
Wound Care Certification Examination**

Dear Future Exam Success Story:

Congratulations on your purchase of our study guide. Our goal in writing our study guide was to cover the content on the test, as well as provide insight into typical test taking mistakes and how to overcome them.

Standardized tests are a key component of being successful, which only increases the importance of doing well in the high-pressure high-stakes environment of test day. How well you do on this test will have a significant impact on your future, and we have the research and practical advice to help you execute on test day.

The product you're reading now is designed to exploit weaknesses in the test itself, and help you avoid the most common errors test takers frequently make.

How to use this study guide

We don't want to waste your time. Our study guide is fast-paced and fluff-free. We suggest going through it a number of times, as repetition is an important part of learning new information and concepts.

First, read through the study guide completely to get a feel for the content and organization. Read the general success strategies first, and then proceed to the content sections. Each tip has been carefully selected for its effectiveness.

Second, read through the study guide again, and take notes in the margins and highlight those sections where you may have a particular weakness.

Finally, bring the manual with you on test day and study it before the exam begins.

Your success is our success

We would be delighted to hear about your success. Send us an email and tell us your story. Thanks for your business and we wish you continued success.

Sincerely,

Mometrix Test Preparation Team

Need more help? Check out our flashcards at: http://MometrixFlashcards.com/WCC

TABLE OF CONTENTS

Top 20 Test Taking Tips

1. Carefully follow all the test registration procedures
2. Know the test directions, duration, topics, question types, how many questions
3. Setup a flexible study schedule at least 3-4 weeks before test day
4. Study during the time of day you are most alert, relaxed, and stress free
5. Maximize your learning style; visual learner use visual study aids, auditory learner use auditory study aids
6. Focus on your weakest knowledge base
7. Find a study partner to review with and help clarify questions
8. Practice, practice, practice
9. Get a good night's sleep; don't try to cram the night before the test
10. Eat a well balanced meal
11. Know the exact physical location of the testing site; drive the route to the site prior to test day
12. Bring a set of ear plugs; the testing center could be noisy
13. Wear comfortable, loose fitting, layered clothing to the testing center; prepare for it to be either cold or hot during the test
14. Bring at least 2 current forms of ID to the testing center
15. Arrive to the test early; be prepared to wait and be patient
16. Eliminate the obviously wrong answer choices, then guess the first remaining choice
17. Pace yourself; don't rush, but keep working and move on if you get stuck
18. Maintain a positive attitude even if the test is going poorly
19. Keep your first answer unless you are positive it is wrong
20. Check your work, don't make a careless mistake

Structures and Functions of Normal Skin

Skin structures

<u>Basement membrane zone</u>
The junction of the epidermis and dermis is the basement membrane zone (BMZ), which provides support for the cells above. It comprises two layers:
- Lamina lucida (because of translucent electrons) contains glycoprotein laminin
- Lamina densa (because of dense electrons) comprises type IV collagen
- Lamina reticularis (bottom portion) is synthesized by cells in connective tissues beneath and contains fibronectin. It contains Type I, II, III and sometimes IV collagen. It serves as the interface between the basement membrane and the underlying connective tissue.

The anchoring structures are composed of hemidesmosomes, which the basal keratocytes use with anchoring filaments and fibrils to attach. BMZ antibodies have been found that react to various antigens. Langerhans cells are part of the immune system. The BMZ is affected by blister formation and disrupted during healing of wounds. The BMZ is modified in skin with psoriasis, affecting adhesion, migration, proliferation and differentiation of keratinocytes, interfering with the normal function of the basement membrane.

<u>Epidermis</u>
The epidermis is the outer avascular layer of skin. It is composed of stratified squamous epithelial cells (keratinocytes) and regenerates every 4-6 weeks:
- Stratum corneum, the outer layer, is flattened dead keratinized cells (corneocytes), providing a waterproof barrier against microorganisms and injury.
- Stratum lucidum is 1-5 translucent cells thick and is found in the palms and soles of the feet where the skin is thicker.
- Stratum granulosum is 1-5 cells thick and contains keratinocytes with granules that contain proteins.
- Stratum spinosum (prickly layers) contains spiny desmosomes that join cube-like cells in multiple layers, providing structure and support.
- Stratum germinativum/stratum basale is one layer of active undifferentiated basal cells with a basement membrane zone beneath. Cells ascend into the stratum spinosum and become keratinocytes. It can take 2-3 weeks for a cell to leave the basal layer and move upward to the stratum corneum, replenishing the various layers. The basal layer contains melanocytes, which provide pigmentation and protection from sunlight.

- 2 -

Dermis and hypodermis
The dermis is the layer beneath the epidermis and BMZ. The dermis contains nerves, sebaceous glands, sweat glands, hair follicles as well as lymphatic vessels, veins and arteries. Fibroblasts produce the primary proteins of this layer, collagen and elastin, with a protein substance called ground substance in the space between them. Mast cells, macrophages, and lymphocytes, which are all involved in the skin immune system (SIS), are also found in the dermis. There are two areas of the dermis:

- Papillary dermis contains the vascular networks that support the epidermis with oxygen and nutrients. It also functions in thermoregulation by regulating blood flow and contains sensory nerve endings.
- Reticular dermis contains the hair follicles and glands and is comprised of connective tissue with collagen and elastic fibers that provides elasticity and strength to the skin. It also contains blood vessels.

The hypodermis comprises the layer of subcutaneous tissue below the dermis, providing vasculature, cushioning, and insulation.

Skin functions

The primary functions of the skin are the following:
- Protection: The skin provides a waterproof barrier to protect against microorganisms, chemicals, and ultraviolet radiation through pigmentation provided by melanocytes.
- Immunity: The skin immune system (SIS) with the Langerhans cells protects against foreign antigens. Mast cells and macrophages destroy pathogenic microorganisms as well as promote tissue repair and wound healing.
- Sensation: The nerve endings are found in the skin, allowing the person to sense pain, pressure, and temperature. Combinations of sensations detected by nerve receptors translate into sensations of burning, itching, and tickling.
- Thermoregulation
- Metabolism: Ultraviolet radiation converts 7-dehydrocholesteral to cholecalciferol, Vitamin D. Vitamin D is synthesized within the skin and then transmits to other parts of the body. It is critical in the metabolism of calcium and phosphate for the formation of bone.
- Appearance: Skin provides a cosmetic appearance and communicates identification

Growth/regeneration in normal skin

Normal skin comprises two layers of tissue (epidermis, dermis) separated by a basement membrane over a layer of subcutaneous tissue (hypodermis). The blood supply that nourishes the growth and regeneration of the skin lies in the subcutaneous tissue and extends into the dermis but not the epidermis, although the blood supplies in the dermis supply nutrients to the epidermis. The epidermis comprises 5 layers: strata corneum, lucidum (extra layer in palms and soles), granulosum, spinosum, and basale. New cells develop and grow in the stratum basale (the deepest layer). As these cells grow, they force the older epidermal cells further away from the dermis toward the outer layers. As the cells move upward, their nutrient supply lessens, and they begin to die. Their cell membranes thicken and harden (keratinization), forming a tough layer of dead cells in the epidermis, the stratum corneum. These cells eventually slough off and are replaced by other dead cells as new cells form below in a continuing cycle of regeneration.

Identification and Management of Risk Factors Impacting Skin Integrity

Pressure ulcers

The Centers for Medicare and Medicaid Services (CMS) established a list of common risk factors for pressure ulcers. Many people present with more than one risk factor. Assessment should include evaluation of risks for following:

- Impairment or decreased mobility or functional ability that prevents a person from changing position.
- Co-morbid conditions affecting circulation or metabolism, such as renal disease, diabetes, and thyroid disease
- Drugs that interfere with healing, such as corticosteroids.
- Impaired circulation, such as generalized atherosclerosis or arterial insufficiency of lower extremity, reducing tissue perfusion.
- Patient refusal of care, increasing risk (positioning, hygiene, nutrition, hydration, skin care).
- Cognitive impairment that prevents patient from reporting discomfort or cooperating with care.
- Fecal and/or urinary contamination of skin, usually related to incontinence.
- Under nutrition or frank malnutrition and/or dehydration.
- Previous healed ulcers. Healed ulcers that were Stage III or IV may deteriorate and breakdown again.

Neuropathic/diabetic ulcers

There are a number of risk factors for the development of neuropathic/ diabetic ulcers:

- Sensory loss can cause sores and ulcers to go undetected in early stages.
- Vascular insufficiency, especially peripheral artery disease occurs 4 times more frequently in diabetics.
- Autonomic neuropathy decreases sweating, leaving feet dry and more prone to cracks and sores.
- Long-term diabetes mellitus with poor glucose control causes severe damage to circulatory system.
- Smoking increases vascular damage and arterial insufficiency.
- Deformities or lack of mobility may increase risk of developing ulcers or having ulcers be undetected.
- Obesity decreases circulation and interferes with control of diabetes. Between 80-90% of diabetics are overweight.
- Male gender increases risk.
- Poor vision may cause people to overlook dangers or prevent them from examining feet and skin.

- Age is associated with increase danger of ulcers.
- Ethnic background can determine genetic risks: Native Americans, Hispanic Americans, African Americans and Pacific Islanders.
- Improperly fitted and supportive footwear can cause ulcerations.

LEAD

There are a number of risk factors for lower extremity arterial disease (LEAD):
- Smoking is a primary cause of LEAD with diagnosis of disease 10 years before non-smokers. It increases the rate of atherosclerosis, decreases HDL, increases blood pressure, and decreases clotting time.
- Obesity raises blood pressure, decreases HDL in cholesterol while raising cholesterol and triglycerides, and increases risk of circulatory disease, including heart attack.
- Lack of exercise decreases pain-free walking distance.

Hypertension correlates with changes in the vessel walls that result in narrowing of blood vessels and decreased circulation.
- Diabetes mellitus causes increased plaque formation, decreased clotting time, increased blood viscosity, and hypertrophy of vasculature. Insulin resistance, related to Type II diabetes increases atherosclerosis. Arterial disease typically progresses faster with diabetes.
- High blood cholesterol, especially LDLs increase atherosclerosis and circulatory impairment.

CVI

There are a number of risk factors for chronic venous insufficiency (CVI) also known as lower-extremity venous disease (LEAD), primarily those that result in valvular dysfunction or calf-muscle dysfunction:
- Obesity with Body Mass Index >25 are more likely to have pressure on pelvic veins, causing valvular dysfunction.
- Intravenous drug use into lower extremities may damage vessels.
- Thrombosis/leg trauma may damage vessels and valves.
- Thrombophlebitis may cause direct damage to valves.
- Thrombophilic conditions, such as protein C deficiency, decrease clotting time of venous blood, increasing risk of thrombosis.
- Varicose veins slow venous return.
- Pregnancy, especially multiple or close pregnancies increase pressure on pelvic veins.
- Lack of exercise/sedentary lifestyle with prolonged periods of sitting result in calf muscle dysfunction.
- Smoking causes vascular changes.

- Age and gender studies show that older women most commonly develop CVI.
- Co-morbid conditions, such as arthritis or those that limit mobility, affect calf-muscle function.

Wound Healing Process

Primary, secondary, and tertiary healing

Primary healing (healing by first intention) involves a wound that is surgically closed by suturing, flaps, or split or full-thickness grafts to completely cover the wound. Primary healing is the most common approach used for surgeries or repair of wounds or lacerations, especially when the wound is essentially "clean." Secondary healing (healing by second intention) involves leaving the wound open and allowing it to close through granulation and epithelialization. Debridement of the wound is done to prepare the wound bed for healing. This approach may be used with contaminated "dirty" or infected wounds to prevent abscess formation and allow the wound to drain. Tertiary healing (healing by third intention) is also sometimes called delayed primary closure because it involves first debriding the wound and allowing it to begin healing while open and then later closing the wound through suturing or grafts. This approach is common with wounds that are contaminated, such as severe animal bites, or wounds related to mixed trauma.

Wound healing phases

There are 4 primary phases to wound healing:
- Hemostasis takes place within the first few minutes after injury and bleeding when the platelets begin to seal off the vessels and secretesubstances that cause vasoconstriction. Thrombin is produced to stimulate the clotting mechanism, forming a fibrin mesh.
- Inflammation (lag or exudative) occurs over days 1-4. During this phase, there is erythema and edema along with pain as the blood vessels release plasma and neutrophils or polymorphonucleocytes to begin phagocytosis to remove debris and prevent infection
- Proliferative/ granulation (fibroblastic) occurs over days 5-20. During this phase, fibroblasts produce collagen to provide support and granulation tissue starts to form. Epithelization occurs and contracture of the wound.
- Maturation (differentiation, remodeling or plateau) occurs after day 21 for an indeterminate duration. The fibroblasts leave the wound and the collagen tightens to reduce scarring. The tissue gains tensile strength. This stage can up to 2 years and the wound can break down easily again during this phase.

Influences on skin's ability to remain intact and/or heal

<u>Age</u>
Age is an important consideration when evaluating the skin because the characteristics of the skin change as people age. An infant 's skin is thinner than an adult's because, while the epidermis is developed, the dermis layer is only about 60% of that of an adult and continues to develop after birth. The skin of premature

infants is especially friable, allowing for transepidermal water loss and evaporative heat loss. During adolescence, the hair follicles activate and the thickness of the dermis decreases about 20% and epidermal turnover time increases, so healing slows. As people continue to age, Langerhans' cells decrease in number, making the skin more prone to cancer, and the inflammatory reactions decrease. The sweat glands, vascularity, and subcutaneous fat all decrease, interfering with thermoregulation and contributing to dryness and irritation of the skin. The epidermal-dermal junction flattens, resulting in skin prone to tearing. The elastin in the skin degrades with age and solar exposure. The thinning of the hypodermis can lead to pressure ulcers.

Sun exposure

Sun exposure is one of the primary factors in aging of the skin, referred to as photoaging or dermatoheliosis. Tanning occurs when ultraviolet radiation (UVR) damages the epidermis and stimulates the production of melanin as a protective mechanism to prevent damage to deeper layers of skin. When the melanin is overpowered, sunburn results, damaging the outer layers of the skin and sometimes the DNA of the skin cells, which can lead to cancer. There are several affects of photoaging that should be noted in assessment:

- Decrease in elasticity and strength.
- Dry, rough, wrinkled skin
- Fine veins on face and ears.
- Freckles and large brown macules (solar lentigines, liver spots) on face, and exposed areas, such as hands and arms and while macules on exposed areas of upper and lower extremities.
- Benign lesions, such as actinic and seborrheic keratoses.
- Malignant lesions, such as basal cell and squamous cell carcinoma.

Lotions, oils, and soaps

Lotions, oils, and soaps all have an affect on the skin. Many oils and lotions are used to increase hydration of the skin. These can include oil baths, which have a minimal effect on hydration but do increase the skin-surface lipids. Lipids are the fatty substances that surround skin cells, and those in the outer layer of skin, the stratum corneum, with fatty acids form the water barrier to retain skin hydration and soften skin. Sebum, produced by the sebaceous glands, is also a lipid. Applying lotion increases the hydration of the epidermis, giving the skin a smoother appearance, and moisturizing lotions also increase the lipids, providing some protection. Alkaline soaps, on the other hand, removes the lipid coating of the skin for about 45 minutes after a normal washing and may increase dryness and susceptibility to bacterial infection. Alcohol and acetone also remove the lipid coating and can increase dehydration of the skin. Acidic cleaners are less irritating than either neutral or alkaline cleaners.

Medications

Medications are a frequent cause of dermatologic effects that can impair the integrity of the skin:

- Photosensitivity can be either photoallergic with exposure to ultraviolet radiation causing an allergic reaction, usually with rash, erythema, edema, and pruritis or phototoxic with the drug being converted into a toxin that causes edema, pain, and pronounced erythema. Thiazide diuretics and conjugated estrogens often cause photosensitive reactions.
- Allergic reactions may involve rash, urticaria or more complex reactions, such as serum sickness. Amoxicillin alone or with clavulanate causes a high rate of these reactions.
- Erythema multiforme has been caused by nifedipine, verapamil, and diltiazem (calcium channel blockers).
- Toxic epidermal necrolysis with full-thickness loss of epidermis can be caused by ranitidine and ciprofloxacin.
- Thinning or atrophy of the skin because of a loss of collagen and telangiectasia (spider veins) are associated with oral, topical, and inhaled corticosteroids.

Management of immunosuppression

Immunosuppression may be the result of co-morbid conditions, such as AIDS, or medications, such as chemotherapy or steroids. Immunosuppression can decrease wound healing and increase the incidence of infection because the body can't destroy pathogenic agents through normal defense mechanisms. Careful management of immunosuppression is critical to healing:

- Adjust dosages or discontinue medications contributing to immunosuppression if possible, including steroid avoidance or steroid withdrawal regimens.
- Monitor wound condition carefully for changes or lack of healing response that may indicate infection because infection is the most common result of immunosuppression and may not be accompanied by increase of temperature or other usual indications.
- Monitor immune status with regular blood tests to determine changes.
- Provide antimicrobials as indicated prophylactically to prevent wound infections.
- Maintain clean environment and ensure staff use standard precautions.
- Observe for opportunistic infections, such as candidiasis.

Glucose control

Management of diabetes and maintaining glucose control for both Type I (insulin-dependent) and Type II diabetes may be the   important determinant of the ability of the wound to heal. Plans should be individualized but usually include the following:
- Establish goals: HbAIC level of 6.5% or lower.
- Maintain normal glycemic levels during healing:
    o Monitor glucose 4 times daily up to every 4 hours.
    o Type I: Monitor food and insulin intake, adjusting as needed.
    o Type II: Focus on diet, medical control, weight loss, and maintenance of weight loss.
    o Avoid or limit use of alcohol because of unpredictable effects on glucose.
- Institute exercise program:
    o Type I: Increases general health and well being.
    o Type II: Decreases insulin resistance.
- Treat co-morbid conditions, such as atherosclerosis, hypertension, and early renal disease.
- Cease smoking, which interferes with circulation and damages vasculature.
- Make lifestyle changes that will promote long-term glucose control.

Control of fecal incontinence

Control of fecal incontinence is necessary to prevent deterioration of tissue that can increase the risk of pressure ulcers and to prevent contamination of existing pressure ulcers:
- Assess incontinence to determine cause and whether it is temporary, related to health problems, or chronic.
- Determine the type of incontinence:
    o Passive, in which the person is unaware.
    o Urge, which is the inability to retain stool.
    o Seepage, after a bowel movement or around a blockage.
- Use medications as indicated to control diarrhea or constipation.
- Place on a bowel-training regimen with scheduled bowel movements using suppositories, stool softeners, bulk formers as indicated, according to cause of incontinence. Use skin moisture barriers and absorbent pads or diapers as needed.
- Modify diet as needed with foods to control diarrhea or constipation.
- Ensure adequate fluid intake.
- Consider fecal pouches or fecal containment devices if incontinence cannot be otherwise controlled.

Control of urinary incontinence

Control of urinary incontinence is necessary to prevent deterioration of the tissue that can increase the risk of pressure ulcers:

- Assess incontinence to determine cause and whether it is temporary, related to health problems, or chronic.
- Temporary Foley catheter may be used in some cases while tissue heals, but long-term use is contraindicated because of the danger of infections.
- Medications may be indicated to treat urinary infections or frequency. Scheduled toileting with reinforcement may help to decrease incidence.
- Use medications as indicated to treat urinary infections or frequency.
- Establish scheduled toileting if indicated.
- Use absorbent pads or adult diapers that wick liquid away from body and establish regular schedule for changing.
- Cleanse soiled skin with no-rinse wipes, as they are less drying to skin than soap and water.
- Use skin moisture barrier ointments to protect skin from urine.

Patient Assessment, Data Collection, and Analysis

Trauma, burns, and infection

Wounds should be evaluated for etiology during the initial assessment to ensure proper treatment. Wounds can arise from a number of different causes:

- Trauma: Injuries resulting from accidents or other types of trauma may vary considerably with some resulting in extensive damage to bones, tissues, organs, and circulation. Additionally, the wounds may be contaminated. Each wound must be assessed individually for multiple factors.
- Burns: Burn wounds may be chemical or thermal and should be assessed according to the area, the percentage of the body burned, and the depth of the burn. First-degree burns are superficial and affect the epidermis. Second-degree burns extend through the dermis. Third degree burns affect underlying tissue, including vasculature, muscles, and nerves.
- Infection: An infected surgical or wound site can result in pain, edema, cellulitis, drainage, erosion of the sutures and ulceration of the tissue. Surgical sites must be assessed carefully and laboratory findings reviewed.

Pressure, arterial, venous stasis, diabetic neuropathy/ischemia

Wounds should be evaluated for etiology during the initial assessment to ensure proper treatment. Wounds can arise from a number of different causes:

- Pressure: Wounds that occur over bony prominences, such as the heels and coccyx, may be related to pressure, shear, or friction. The skin should be carefully examined for discolorations or changes in texture that might indicate compromise.
- Arterial: Arterial insufficiency is associated with decrease in pedal pulse, cool atrophic (shiny, dry) skin. It may result in small punctate-type ulcers, frequently on the dorsum of foot.
- Venous stasis: A decrease in venous circulation often results in hemoglobin leaking into the tissues of the lower leg, giving a brown discoloration. Tissue is often edematous, and ulcers are most common near the medial malleolus.
- Diabetic neuropathy/ischemia: Neuropathy can result in lack of sensation to pain so that injuries to feet may go unnoticed. Diabetes may also cause damage to small vessels, resulting in ischemia that can lead to ulcerations.

Subtle indications of infection with arterial insufficiency

Because of the lack of circulation, the normal signs of inflammation and infection may be evident with arterial insufficiency, so observing for subtle signs of infection is critically important. Prompt identification and treatment is necessary to prevent cellulitis and/or osteomyelitis that may result in amputation. Dry necrotic wounds should be painted with 10% povidone-iodine and covered with dry gauze, but the ulcer and the skin around should be inspected daily. Indications of infection include:

- Increased pain in the ischemic limb or ulcer and/or increased edema.
- Increase in necrotic area of ulcer.
- Periwound tissue has fluctuance evident on palpation (soft wave-like texture) that may indicate infection in the tissue.
- Erythema about the perimeter of the wound may be very slight.

At any indication of infection, culture and sensitivities should be done so that appropriate therapy can begin.

Lymphedema

Lymphedema is a dysfunction of the lymphatic system, resulting in a debilitating progressive disease. The healthy lymphatic system returns proteins, lipids, and fluids to the circulatory system from the interstitial spaces, but with lymphedema this accumulates, causing pronounced induration, edema, and fibrosis of tissues. As the fluid builds up, it causes distention, and the skin becomes thick and fibrotic with orange discoloration (pea d'orange). Scaly keratinic debris collects, and the skin develops cracks and leakage of lymphatic fluid. Lymphedema may be primary (developmental abnormality) or secondary. It can occur after mastectomy and after radiation, infection, cancer or surgery, such as joint replacements and vascular procedures. Patients are at risk of infection, cellulitis and lymphangitis, as well as pain and limited mobility. Lymphedema has 3 stages:

- Stage 1 is reversible pitting edema distally with no fibrosis.
- Stage 2 is pitting or non-pitting edema with fibrosis and papillomatosis.
- Stage 3 is elephantiasis with massive enlargement and distortion of limb, fibrosis and ulcerations.

Diagnostic testing

Total protein and albumin
Total protein levels can be influenced by many factors, including stress and infection, but it may be monitored as part of an overall nutritional assessment. Protein is critical for wound healing, and because metabolic rate increases in response to a wound, protein needs increase:

- Normal values: 5-9g/kL.
- Diet requirements for wound healing: 1.25-1.5 g/kg per day.

Albumin is a protein that is produced by the liver and is a necessary component for cells and tissues. Levels decrease with renal disease, malnutrition, and severe burns. Albumin levels are the most common screening to determine protein levels. Albumin has a half-life of 18-20 days, so it is sensitive to long-term protein deficiencies more than short-term.

- Normal values: 3.5-5.5 g/dL
- Mild deficiency: 3-3.5 g/dL
- Moderate deficiency: 2.5-3.0 g/dL
- Severe deficiency: <2.5 g/dL.

Levels below 3.2 correlate with increased morbidity and death. Dehydration (poor intake, diarrhea, or vomiting) elevates levels, so adequate hydration is important to ensure meaningful results

Transferrin
Transferrin, which transports about one-third of the body's iron, is a protein produced by the liver. It transports iron from the intestines to the bone marrow where it is used to produce hemoglobin. The half-life of transferrin is about 8-10 days. It is sometimes used as a measure of nutritional status; however, transferrin levels are sensitive to many different things. Levels rapidly decrease with protein malnutrition. Liver disease and anemia can also depress levels, but a decrease in iron, commonly found with inadequate protein, stimulates the liver to produce more transferrin, which increases levels but also decreases production of albumin and prealbumin. Levels may also increase with pregnancy, use of oral contraceptives, and polycythemia. Thus, transferrin levels alone are not always reliable measurements of nutritional status:

- Normal values: 200-400 mg/dL.
- Mild deficiency: 150-200 mg/dL.
- Moderate deficiency: 100-150 mg/dL.
- Severe deficiency: <100 mg/dL.

Prealbumin
Prealbumin (transthyretin) is most commonly monitored for acute changes in nutritional status because it has a half-life of only 2-3 days. Prealbumin is a protein produced in the liver, so it is often decreased with liver disease. Oral contraceptives and estrogen can also decrease levels. Levels may rise with Hodgkin's disease or the use of steroids or NSAIDS. Prealbumin is necessary for transportation of both thyroxine and vitamin A throughout the body, so if levels fall, both thyroxine and vitamin A utilization are also affected.

- Normal values: 16-40 mg/dL.
- Mild deficiency: 10-15mg/dL
- Moderate deficiency: 5-9 mg/dL.
- Severe deficiency: <5 mg/dL.

Prealbumin is a good measurement because it quickly decreases when nutrition is inadequate and rises quickly in response to increased protein intake. Protein intake must be adequate to maintain levels of prealbumin. Death rates increase with any decrease in prealbumin levels.

Total lymphocyte count

The immune system responds quickly to changes in protein intake because proteins are critical to antibody and lymphocyte production. T lymphocytes develop in the thymus gland and are a part of the cell-mediated immune response. B-lymphocytes develop in the bone marrow and are part of the humoral (antibody-mediated) immune response. Total lymphocyte count (TLC) can reflect changes in nutritional status because a decrease in protein causes decreased immunity. Lymphocytes are expressed on a differential as a percentage of the white blood count. The TLC is calculated by multiplying the percentage by the total white blood count and then dividing by 100.

- Normal values: 2000 cells/mm^3.
- Mild deficiency: 1500-1800 cells/mm^3.
- Moderate deficiency: 900-1500 cells/mm^3.
- Severe deficiency: <900 cells/mm^3.

While low levels may be indicative of malnutrition, levels are also depressed with stress, autoimmune diseases, chemotherapy, infection, and HIV.

Glucose and Hemoglobin AIC

Glucose is manufactured by the liver from ingested carbohydrates and is stored as glycogen for use by the cells. If intake is inadequate, glucose can be produced from muscle and fat tissue, leading to increased wasting. High levels of glucose are indicative of diabetes mellitus, which predisposes people to skin injuries, slow healing, and infection. Fasting blood glucose levels are used to diagnose and monitor:

- Normal values: 70-99 mg/dL. Impaired: 100-125 mg/dL.
- Diabetes: $\geq$126 mg/dL.

There are a number of different conditions that can increase glucose levels: stress, renal failure, Cushing syndrome, hyperthyroidism, and pancreas disorders. Medications, such as steroids, estrogens, lithium, phenytoin, diuretics, tricyclic antidepressants, may increase glucose levels. Other conditions, such as adrenal insufficiency, liver disease, hypothyroidism, and starvation can decrease glucose levels. Hemoglobin AIC comprises hemoglobin A with a glucose molecule because hemoglobin holds onto excess blood glucose, so it shows the average blood glucose levels over a 2-3 month period and is used primarily to monitor long-term diabetic therapy.

- Normal value: $\leq$6%
- Elevation: >7%

Complete blood count with WBCs and differential

White blood cell (leukocyte) count is used as an indicator of bacterial and viral infection. WBC is reported as the total number of all white blood cells.

- Normal WBC for adults: 4,800-10,000
- Acute infection: 10,000+; 30,000 indicates a severe infection.
- Viral infection: 4,000 and below

The differential provides the percentage of each different type of leukocyte. An increase in the white blood cell count is usually related to an increase in one type and often an increase in immature neutrophils, known as bands, referred to as a "shift to the left, an indication of an infectious process:

- Normal immature neutrophils (bands): 1-3%. Increase with infection
- Normal segmented neutrophils (segs) for adults: 50-62%. Increase with acute, localized, or systemic bacterial infections.
- Normal eosinophils: 0-3%. Decrease with stress and acute infection.
- Normal basophils: 0-1%. Decrease during acute stage of infection.
- Normal lymphocytes; 25-40%. Increase in some viral and bacterial infections.
- Normal monocytes: 3-7%. Increase during recovery stage of acute infection.

Complete blood count with RBCs, platelets, Hgb and Hct

The complete blood count with differential and platelet (thrombocyte) count provides information about the blood and other body systems. Red blood cell (erythrocyte) counts and concentrations may vary with anemia, hemorrhage or various disorders and decrease may affect healing because of less oxygen to tissues, but changes do not indicate infection.

Hemoglobin, a protein found in erythrocytes, uses iron to bind and transport oxygen. Deficiencies of amino acids, vitamins or minerals can cause a decrease, impacting healing and increasing the danger of pressure ulcers by reducing oxygen to tissue. Dehydration and severe burns can cause an increase.

- Normal values: Males, 13-18 g/dL. Females, 12-16 g/dL.

Hematocrit measures the percentage of packed red blood cells in 100 ml of blood. A decrease can indicate blood loss and anemia. An increase may indicate dehydration, and measurements may monitor the effects of rehydration.

- Normal values: Males, 42-52%. Females, 37-48%.

Platelet normal values of 150,000-400,000 may increase to over a million during acute infection.

C-reactive protein and erythrocyte sedimentation rate

C-reactive protein is an acute-phase reactant produced by the liver in response to an inflammatory response that causes neutrophils, granulocytes and macrophages to secrete cytokines. Thus, levels of C-reactive protein rise when there is inflammation or infection. It has been found to be helpful to measure of response to treatment for pyoderma gangrenosum ulcers:

- Normal values: 2.6-7.6 µg/dL.

Erythrocyte sedimentation rate (sed rate) measures the distance erythrocytes fall in a vertical tube of anticoagulated blood in one hour. Because fibrinogen, which increases in response to infection, slows the fall, the sed rate can be used as a non-specific test for inflammation when infection is suspected. The sed rate is sensitive to osteomyelitis and may be used to monitor treatment response. Values vary according to gender and age:

- <50: Males 0-15 mm/hr. Females 0-20 mm/hr.
- >50: Males 0-20 mm/hr. Females 0-30 mm/hr.

Wound culture

Wound culture and sensitivities are done when there are signs of infection in a wound or no progress in healing over a two-week period. The wound culture identifies the pathogenic agent and the sensitivities show which antimicrobials are the most affective for treatment. The culture should be done prior to the administration of antibiotics, which may interfere with the results. Sterile technique should be used. A culture area may be done, taking the sample from clean tissue rather than exudate, which may give a false report, showing organisms in the area but not in the tissue itself. There are 3 methods of culturing:

- Swabbing the area is the most common method used but the sample is easily contaminated by surface flora.
- Needle aspiration of fluid adjacent to the wound may result in underestimation of organisms.
- Culturing by tissue biopsy is often most effective method, but not all labs can process these samples and the process disrupts the wound and increases pain.

Diagnostic testing for hydration

Serum sodium and osmolality

Hydration is essential for proper healing and for meaningful results of laboratory measures of nutrition. A number of different tests can be used to monitor hydration. Serum sodium measures the sodium level in the blood. Some drugs, such as steroids, laxatives, contraceptives, NSAIDS, and IV fluids containing sodium can elevate levels. Other drugs, such as diuretics and vasopressin can reduce levels.

- Normal values: 135-150 mEq/L.
- Dehydration: >150 mE/L.

Serum osmolality measures the concentration of ions, such as sodium, chloride, potassium, glucose, and urea in the blood. Levels increase with dehydration, which stimulates the antidiuretic hormone (AD), resulting in increased water reabsorption and more concentrated urine in an effort to compensate. Changes in osmolality can affect normal cell functioning, eventually destroying the cells if levels remain high.

- Normal levels: 285-295 mill-osmoles per kilogram/ H_2O.
- Dehydration: >295 mOsm/kg H_2O.

BUN, BUN-creatinine ratio, and specific gravity/urine

A number of different tests can be used to monitor hydration:
- Blood urea nitrogen (BUN), a protein by-product, is excreted by the kidneys. An elevation of both BUN and creatinine indicates kidney disease, but elevated BUN alone may indicate dehydration:
  - Normal values: 7-23 mg/dl.
  - Dehydration: >23 mg/dl.
- BUN-creatinine ratio monitors renal failure, where there is enhanced reabsorption in the proximal tubules, causing the urea level to rise. Dehydration or conditions that limit fluid into the kidneys increases urea. Increased urea is also an indication of an upper GI bleed where the proteins in the blood are broken down and reabsorbed in the lower intestinal tract.
  - Normal value: 10:1
  - Dehydration: >25:1.
- Specific gravity/urine measures the ability of the kidneys to concentrate or dilute the urine according to changes in serum. The most common cause of an increased specific gravity is dehydration. It may also increase with an increased secretion of anti-diuretic hormone (ADH).
  - Normal value: 1.003-1.028
  - Dehydration: >1.028

Triceps skinfold thickness, mid-arm circumference, and mid-arm muscle circumference

Triceps skinfold thickness is measured using special calipers. The midpoint between the axilla and elbow of the non-dominant arm is measured and located and then the skin is grasped about 1 cm above the midpoint between the thumb and index finger by grasping at the edges of the arm and moving the finger and thumb inward until a firm fold of tissue is observed. The calipers are placed about this fold at the midpoint (right below the fingers) and squeezed for 3 seconds and then a measurement is taken to the nearest millimeter. Three readings are taken with the average of the three used as the measurement. Mid-arm circumference (MAC) measurement is obtained by measuring in centimeters at the midpoint between the axilla and elbow. Mid-arm muscle circumference (MAMC) is calculated by multiplying the triceps skinfold thickness (in millimeters) by *pi* (3.14), and subtracting the result from the midarm circumference with results in centimeters.

Triceps skinfold thickness (TST) evaluates fat stores, which often change slowly, so this is not a sensitive test for malnutrition, but it can be used to determine if fat is increasing while muscle mass is decreasing. Mid-arm circumference (MAC) measures muscles, bones, and skin and mid-arm muscle circumference (MAMC) measures lean body mass. These vary considerably between individuals so are more useful to track muscle wasting over time than for comparisons. The TST, MAC, and MAMC are recorded as a percentage of standard measurements, which are quantified for males and females.

- Males
  - TST 12.5 mm
  - MAC 29.9 cm
  - MAMC 25.3 cm
- Females
  - TST 16.5 mm
  - MAC 28.5 cm
  - MAMC 23.3 cm

In order to reach the percentage, the actual measurement for each test is divided by the standard measurement and that result in multiplied by 100. Thus, if a male's TST measured 11.8:

$$11.8 \div 12.5 = 0.944 \times 100 = 94.4\%$$

BMI

The Body Mass Index (BMI) I formula is a measurement that uses height and weight as an indicator of obesity/malnutrition. This cannot be used alone to diagnose obesity as body types differ considerably. Women often have more body fat than men. Tables are available to make calculations simple, but the BMI can be calculated manually:

BMI formula using pounds and inches:

$$BMI = \frac{(\text{weight in pounds} \times 703)}{\text{Height in inches}^2}$$

BMI formula using kilograms and meters:

$$BMI = \frac{\text{weight in kilograms}}{\text{Height in meters}^2}$$

Resulting scores for adults age 20 and over are interpreted according to this chart:

- Below 18.5 Underweight
- 18.5-24.9 Normal weight
- 25.0-29.9 Overweight
- 30 and above Obese

BMI for those under age 20 uses age-gender specific charts provided by the CDC, containing a curved line that indicates percentiles. The criteria for obesity based on these charts and BMI for age are as follows:

- <5th percentile Underweight
- 85th-<95 percentile At risk for overweight
- ≥95th percentile Overweight

Waist Hip Ratio

The Waist Hip Ratio (WHR) is the ratio of fat stored about the abdomen and the fat stored around the hips. This ratio is considered of increasing import because an increase in this ratio is associated with increased risk of heart disease, brain attacks, and diabetes mellitus. The formula:

$$WHR = \frac{\text{waist circumference in centimeters}}{\text{Hip circumference in centimeters}}$$

The waist measurement is taken at the smallest circumference, usually slightly above the umbilicus, and the hip measurement at the widest part of the hips, usually about 7 inches below the waist. The results of the calculation provide a score with risks according to gender:

- Males >1 = increased risk
- Females   >0.85 = increased risk

Studies have indicated that people who care more weight around their waists relative to their hips (apple-shaped) are more at risk for complications related to weight than those that carry more weight in their hips (pear-shaped).

Measuring head circumference to assess nutrition

Head circumference measurements are taken for children during the first 3 years. While there can be non-nutritional reasons for decreased growth of the head, it can also be a sign of severe lack of nutrition and may be associated with decreased linear growth as well. The procedure:

- Use non-stretchable measuring tape.
- Child should be standing or held in sitting position with head upright.
- Place tape around head just above the eyebrows in the font and around the occipital area in the back.
- Take at least 3 readings or more until 2 measurements are within 0.1 cm.
- Use growth chart to determine if measurement is within normal limits.

The CDC provides growth charts for both head circumference and linear growth that are specific for gender, showing the percentile ranking of measurements. Evaluation depends upon various factors, including results of height and weight measurement, to determine if a child is undernourished although findings below the 5th percentile are usually cause for concern.

ABI

The ankle-brachial index (ABI) examination is done to evaluate peripheral arterial disease of the lower extremities.

- Apply blood pressure cuff to one arm, palpate brachial pulse, and place conductivity gel over the artery.
- Place the tip of a Doppler device at a 45-degree angle into the gel at the brachial artery and listen for the pulse sound.
- Inflate the cuff until the pulse sound ceases and then inflate 20mm Hg above that point.
- Release air and listen for the return of the pulse sound. This reading is the brachial systolic pressure.
- Repeat the procedure on the other arm, and use the higher reading for calculations.
- Repeat the same procedure on each ankle with the cuff applied above the malleoli and the gel over they posterior tibial pulse to obtain the ankle systolic pressure.
- Divide the ankle systolic pressure by the brachial systolic pressure to obtain the ABI.

Sometimes, readings are taken both before and after 5 minutes of walking on a treadmill.

Once the ankle-brachial index (ABI) examination is completed, the ankle systolic pressure must be divided by the brachial systolic pressure. Ideally, the blood pressure at the ankle should be equal to that of the arm or slightly higher. With peripheral arterial disease, the ankle pressure falls, affecting the ABI. Additionally, some conditions that cause calcification of arteries, such as diabetes, can cause a false elevation. Calculation is simple; if the ankle systolic pressure is 90 and the brachial systolic pressure is 120:

$$90 \div 120 = .75$$

The degree of disease relates to the score:
- >1.3 Abnormally high, may indicate calcification of vessel wall
- 1-1.1: Normal reading, asymptomatic
- <0.95 Indicates narrowing of one or more leg blood vessels
- <0.8 Moderate, often associated with intermittent claudication during exercise
- ≤ 0.6-0.8 Borderline perfusion
- 0.5-0.75 Severe disease, ischemia,
- <0.5 Pain even at rest, limb threatened
- 0.25 Critical limb-threatening condition

TBI

The procedure and interpretation of results of Toe-brachial index (TBI) are explained below:

- Apply blood pressure cuff to one arm, palpate brachial pulse, and place conductivity gel over the artery.
- Place the tip of a Doppler device at a 45-degree angle into the gel at the brachial artery and listen for the pulse sound.
- Inflate the cuff until the pulse sound ceases and then inflate 20mm Hg above that point.
- Release air and listen for the return of the pulse sound. This reading is the brachial systolic pressure.
- Repeat the procedure on the other arm, and use the higher reading for calculations.
- Repeat the same procedure on the great or second toe with the cuff applied around the base of the toes and the gel over the pulse to obtain the toe systolic pressure.
- Divide the toe systolic pressure by the brachial systolic pressure to obtain the TBI (same calculations as for ABI). Normal values are >0.6.

Transcutaneous oxygen pressure measurement

Transcutaneous oxygen pressure measurement ($TCPO_2$) is a non-invasive test that measures dermal oxygen, showing effectiveness of oxygen in the skin and tissues. Contact gel and electrodes are applied to the lower extremities to determine variations in oxygen tension. The electrodes are placed in special fixation rings attached to the skin to prevent environment air from affecting the readings, and then the skin is heated to increase blood flow. Two or three different sites should be tested to give a more accurate demonstration of oxygenation. This test is used for a number of purposes:

- Determining if there is enough oxygen transport for effective hyperbaric oxygen therapy treatments.
- Determining the degree of oxygenation and peripheral vascular disease.
- Establishing the degree of hypoxia in venous diseases.
- Identifying the optimum site for amputation of severely hypoxic limbs.

Test results:
- >40 mm Hg adequate oxygenation for healing.
- 20-40 mm Hg equivocal finding.
- <20 mm Hg marked ischemia, affecting healing.

Multidisciplinary consultation

A multidisciplinary team is comprised of experts in a number of different fields, collaborating to address the complex problems associated with wound care and underlying pathology. Instead of the serial approach to problem solving involved in the traditional model of care, where referrals are made in response to problems that arise with little communication among specialists, the multidisciplinary approach is to identify potential problems and institute preventive measure at the onset with all members communicating and sharing information. Responsibilities of the wound care team include:

- Prevention: Establish standard risk assessment protocols and formulary. Incorporate national prevention guidelines.
- Treatment: Establish clinical protocols and product formularies in relation to national treatment practice guidelines.
- Documentation: Provide standardized methods.
- Education: Provide literature/training for patients and staff/
- Quality Management: Evaluate outcomes and disseminate findings
- Research: Conduct clinical trials
- Care conferences: Create individualized care plans.

Referrals for medical/surgical interventions

Referrals for medical surgical interventions are an important part of wound care as healing requires that medical conditions be monitored carefully and treated, especially such disorders as diabetes and peripheral vascular disease, but this is also true of almost all acute or chronic disorders. Conditions that were stable prior to wound development may deteriorate or change in character in response to the body's needs during healing or infections that may occur. Patients may require referrals, such as to endocrinologists or infectious disease specialists. Wounds with extensive eschar may require surgical debridement in order to promote healing. It is important that the patient be an integral member of any planning and discussion. The patient must be apprised of the reasons for referrals and the types of testing, care, and procedures that will be done to ensure cooperation and to alleviate patient's fears and anxiety.

Identification of patient goals and factors affecting care

It's easy to confuse nursing goals with patient goals. Nursing goals involve restoring a patient to the best health possible; however, patients' goals may be very different, or patients may lack defined goals. The only way to help patients to establish goals is to talk to them, helping them arrive at realistic short-term and long-term goals based on their condition and abilities. There are a number of factors that can affect goals and care:

- Functional disability may prevent a patient from taking the steps needed to reach a goal.
- Mental status may be such that a patient is not competent to set goals or to carry out needed actions.
- Co-morbidity may result in health problems that interfere with plan of care.
- Low income may prevent a patient from buying supplies or getting needed assistance.
- Social circumstances may be such that the patient lacks family support or is dependent on others.
- Smoking may impact healing.

Assessment of edema

Edema is usually checked by pressing the index finger into the tissue on top of each foot, behind the medial malleolus, and over the shin, starting distally and moving proximally to the highest level of edema, comparing both legs:

- Edema is rated on a 1-4 point scale:
    - 1+ slight pitting to about 2 mm (persists 10-15 seconds).
    - 2+ moderate pitting to about 4 mm (persists 10-15 seconds).
    - 3+ moderate-severe pitting to about 6 mm (persists >1 minute).
    - 4+ severe pitting to 8 mm or more (persists 2-5 minutes).
- Venous edema: edema from ankle to knee and may involve some limitation in ankle movement. Dependent pitting edema occurs, but may become non-pitting in chronic disease.
- Lymphedema: usually unilateral non-pitting hard edema from toes to groin. In advanced disease, elephantiasis with huge enlargement of extremity may occur.
- Lipedema: symmetrical bilateral soft rubbery tissue from ankle to groin and sometimes hips with pain on palpation and frequent bruising.

Norton assessment tool

The Norton assessment tool (Norton scale) (1961) was originally devised to evaluate the risk of pressure sores, although it provides less accurate risk assessment than some newer scales like the Braden scale. However, the ease of use of the Norton scale is an advantage. The Norton scale comprises 5 subscales, each rated on a scale of 1 to 4:
- Physical condition: (4) good, (3) fair, (2) bad, (2) very bad.
- Mental state: (4) alert, (3) apathetic, (2) confused, (1) stuporous.
- Activity: (4) ambulatory, (3) assisted walking, (2) chair-bound, (1) bedridden.
- Mobility: (4) full, (3) slightly impaired, (2) very limited, (1) immobile.
- Incontinence: (4) none, (3) occasional, (2) usually urinary, (1) urinary and fecal.

The scores are added together to arrive at a final score with lower scores indicating risk:
- 18 to 20: Low risk
- 14 to 17: Medium risk
- 10 to 13: High risk
- ≤9: Very high risk

Braden scale

The Braden scale is a risk assessment tool that has been validated clinically as predictive of the risk of patient's developing pressure sores. It was developed in 1988 by Barbara Braden and Nancy Bergstrom and is in wide use. The scale scores 6 different areas with 1-4 points.
- Sensory perception:
  - 1.- Completely limited (unresponsive to pain or limited ability to feel)
  - 2.- Very limited (responds to painful stimuli and moans)
  - 3.- Slightly limited (responds to verbal commands but limited communication)
  - 4.- No impairment
- Moisture:
  - 1.- Moist constantly
  - 2.- Very moist (linen change each shift)
  - 3.- Occasionally moist (linen change each day)
  - 4.- Rarely moist
- Activity:
  - 1.- Bed bound
  - 2.- Chair bound
  - 3.- Walks occasionally (short distances)
  - 4.- Walks frequently

- Mobility:
  - 1.- Completely immobile
  - 2.- Very limited (makes occasional slight position changes)
  - 3.- Slightly limited (makes frequently slight position changes)
  - 4.- No limitations
- Usual nutrition pattern:
  - 1.- Very poor (eats < half of meals inadequate protein, intake, and hydration)
  - 2.- Inadequate (eats about 1/2 of food with 3 protein serving or not enough liquid or tube feeding)
  - 3.- Adequate (eats > half of meals and 4 protein servings)
  - 4.- Excellent
- Friction and shear (3 parameters only):
  - 1.- Problem moving (skin frequently slides down sheets, needs help to move)
  - 2.- Potential problem (moves weakly or needs some assistance, skin slides somewhat during moves)
  - 3.- No apparent problem.

The scores for all six items are totaled and a risk assigned according to the number:
- 23 (best score) excellent prognosis, very minimal risk
- ≤ 16 breakpoint for risk of pressure ulcer (will vary somewhat for different populations)
- 6 (worst score) prognosis is very poor, strong likelihood of developing pressure ulcer.

PUSH assessment tool

The National Pressure Ulcer Advisory Panel (NPUAP) developed the Pressure Ulcer Scale for Healing (PUSH) tool to aid in the assessment of pressure ulcers over time. The scale comprises 3 subscales:
- Surface area (length X width in cm^2): Scored 0 (healed) to 1(<0.3 cm) to 10 (>24.0 cm). Measure the greatest length by greatest width using a centimeter ruler.
- Amount of exudate: Scored 0 (none), 1 (light), 2 (moderate), or 3 (heavy).
- Tissue type: Scored 0 (closed, 1 (epithelial), 2 (granulation), 3 (slough), or 4 (necrotic). Necrotic tissue is black/brown and crusted; slough, yellow or white tissue; granulation, moist granular pink or beefy red; and epithelial, pink or shiny.

The scores for the 3 subscales are added together and the total scores tabulated for comparison to determine if the ulcer is healing or deteriorating. Scores may also be graphed for a visual representation.

Nylon monofilament test

A simple test for neuropathy, commonly used to determine risk of ulcers in diabetic patients, is the nylon monofilament test, which is available in kits:

- Describe the procedure to the patient and ask the patient to indicate when the pressure of the monofilament is felt.
- Grasp a length of #10 monofilament in the instrument provided.
- Touch the monofilament against the bottom of the foot and then press the monofilament into the foot until the line buckles.
- Test the great, 3rd, and 5th toes.
- Test the left, medial, and right areas of the ball of the foot
- Test the right and left of the arch.
- Test the middle of the heel.

The test is evaluated according to how many of the 10 test sites the patient is able to detect. If the patient fails to detect the monofilament at fewer than 4 sites, this is indicative of decreased sensation and increased risk.

Assessment of lower extremities

Assessment of lower extremities includes a number of different elements:

- Appearance includes comparing limbs for obvious differences or changes in skin or nails as well as evaluating for edema, color changes in skin, such as pallor or rubor. Legs that are thin, pale, shiny, and hairless indicate peripheral arterial disease.
- Perfusion should be assessed by checking venous filling time and capillary refill, skin temperature (noting changes in one limb or between limbs), bruits (indicating arterial narrowing), pulses (comparing both sides in a proximal to distal progression), ankle-brachial index and toe-brachial index.
- Sensory function includes the ability to feel pain, temperature, and touch.
- Range of motion of the ankle must be assessed to determine if the joint flexes past 90° because this is necessary for unimpaired walking and aids venous return in the calf.
- Pain is an important diagnostic feature of peripheral arterial disease, so the location, intensity, duration, and characteristics of pain are important.

Evaluation of the pulses of the lower extremities is an important part of assessment for peripheral arterial disease. *Pulses* should be first evaluated with the patient in supine position and then again with the legs dependent, checking bilaterally and proximally to distally to determine if intensity of pulse decreases distally. Pedal pulses should be examined at both the posterior tibialis and the dorsalis pedis. The pulse should be evaluated as to the rate, rhythm, and intensity, which is usually graded on a 0-4 scale:

- pulse absent
- weak, difficult to palpate

- normal as expected
- full
- strong and bounding

Pulses may be palpable or absent with peripheral arterial disease. Absence of pulse on both palpation and Doppler probe does indicate peripheral arterial disease. *Bruits* may be noted by auscultating over major arteries, such as femoral, popliteal, peroneal, and dorsalis pedis, indicating peripheral arterial disease.

> ➤ **Review Video:** <u>Range of Motion Therapy</u>
> *Visit **mometrix.com/academy** and enter **Code:** **191142***

Assessing perfusion of lower extremities

Assessment of perfusion can indicate venous or arterial abnormalities:
- Venous refill time: Begin with the patient lying supine for a few moments and then have the patient sit with the feet dependent. Observe the veins on the dorsum of the foot and count the seconds before normal filling. Venous occlusion is indicated with times >20 seconds.
- Capillary refill: Grasp the toenail bed between the thumb and index finger and apply pressure for several seconds to cause blanching. Release the nail and count the seconds until the nail regains normal color. Arterial occlusion is indicated with times >2-3 seconds. Checks both feet and more than one nail bed.
- Skin temperature: Using the palm of the hand and fingers, gently palpate the skin, moving distally to proximally and comparing both legs. Arterial disease is indicated by decreased temperature (coolness) or a marked change from proximal to distal. Venous disease is indicated by increased temperature about the ankle.

Skin changes and abnormalities LEVD

Skin changes and abnormalities, in addition to edema, related to lower-extremity venous disease (LEVD include:
- Hemosiderin staining occurs when hemosiderin, a brownish granular iron-containing pigment resulting from breakdown of hemoglobin, builds up in the interstitial fluid as a result of venous hypertension causing the erythrocytes to seep into the tissues. As the cells break down, the deposits along with melanin remain in the tissue. This causes a brownish, splotchy discoloration of the skin from the ankle to the anterior tibial area.
- Lipodermatosclerosis occurs in the lower leg area as the tissue becomes fibrotic from fibrin and protein (collagen) deposits, causing the skin to feel waxy and the tissue to harden with narrowing of the tissue around the ankle compared to proximal tissue above.

- Venous (stasis) dermatitis is inflammation of the epidermis and dermis resulting in scaly, erythematous, crusty, weepy, itchy skin, usually in the lower leg (ankle and tibia). It is progressive with redness and itching appearing before other symptoms.
- Malleolar flare is caused by capillaries in a sunburst pattern inferior and distal to the medial malleolus.
- Atropie blanche lesions are smooth white avascular sclerotic skin plaques that occur in about one-third of patients with LEVD. They are usually associated with torturous vessels and hemosiderin staining on the ankles or foot. They may appear similar to scarring from healed ulcers but actually have a high risk for deteriorating into ulcer formation.
- Varicosities (varicose veins) are veins where blood has pooled, causing them to become distended, twisted, and palpable, often appearing as blue rope-like vessels on back of the knee and calf or inside of the leg. They are the result of venous reflux and venous hypertension.
- Ankle blowout syndrome occurs when small vessels around the medial malleolus, creating a number of small very painful ulcers.

Assessment of LEND leading to neuropathic/diabetic wounds

The assessment for lower extremity neuropathic disease (LEND) and neuropathic/diabetic wounds includes:
- History: A history of general health and record of diabetes control and complications is critical. Risk factors should be identified and risks classified according to severity.
- Physical examination: The examination must identify any co-morbid conditions, such as heart disease, arthritis, and peripheral arterial or venous insufficiency.
- Lower extremity/foot examination: A thorough examination of the lower extremity and foot should include screening for neuropathy and sensory loss, pain, musculoskeletal changes or abnormalities, and vascular status. The skin should be carefully assessed for corns, calluses, pre-ulcerative lesions (such as blisters or cracks). Nails should be checked for fungus infections and thickening, which is common, and discolorations, such as red, black, or brown that may indicate trauma. Footwear should be examined for support and fit.
- Evaluation and classification of the diabetic foot ulcer (DFU): Ulcers should be measured and classified according to standard classification systems, observing for signs of infection.

Assessment for foot deformities related to diabetic ulcers

- Inflammation of connective tissue from the heel to ball of foot:
    - Plantar fasciitis causes severe heel pain.
- Bony heel growths
    - Heel spurs are abnormal protruding growths of bone on the calcaneus, leading to plantar fascitis.
- Distal muscle atrophy
    - Hammer toe (contracture of proximal joint of toe)
    - Mallet toe (contracture of distal joint of toe)
    - Claw toe (contracture of both joints of toe)
- Changes in metatarsal bones
    - Metatarsal bones lower or longer than adjoining bones uneven weight distribution, resulting in pain and ulceration.
    - Bunion (enlargement of first metatarsal bone below first toe).
- Arch changes
    - High cramped instep (*pes cavus*)
    - Flat foot (*pes covus*)
- Weakening of dorsum/plantar surfaces.
    - Charcot's arthropathy involves weakened bones fracturing and the foot changing shape and becoming inflamed as the arch collapses, causing the foot to have a convex shape.
- Nerve irritation
    - Neuromas between toes.

Assessment of wounds at the end-of-life

While the primary goals of skin care are to prevent and heal wounds, when patients near the end-of-life there are a number of issues to assess:
- Hospice care
- Advance directives
- Best interests of patient

Patients under hospice care are to receive palliative rather than curative treatment, but in the case of wound care, sometimes treatments that are essentially curative are appropriate if they reduce pain and discomfort. The Patient Self-determination Act allows people to refuse treatment when they are competent to make that decision and to make advance directives about end-of-life care, and this must be respected in relation to wound care. As the systems deteriorate near the end of life, these patients are prone to pressure sores, so deciding what must be treated and what treatment is futile can be difficult. Frequently changing the patient's position to prevent pressure may increase pain and discomfort. These decisions must be individualized.

Assessing activities in relation to pain

Assessment of pain must include determining those factors or activities that increase pain.

- Site of pain: While pain is often focused on the wound site, it may extend to the surrounding tissues, especially in chronic wounds, making application and removal of dressings especially painful.
- Movement: Pressure and touch caused by changes of position can increase pain, limiting mobility.
- Time: Pain often increases at night, making sleep difficult.
- Dressings: Dressings that are too tight or the wrong choice for a wound may cause intense site pain. Allowing the wound to become dry can also increase pain.
- Personal/ cultural: Some people have difficulty expressing the degree of pain. Others react to the expectation of the medical personnel or family. Some believe that they should remain stoic or are afraid of becoming "addicted" and resist taking pain medications until pain is severe.

Pain assessment

Pain is subjective and may be influenced by the individual's pain threshold (the smallest stimulus that produces the sensation of pain) and pain tolerance (the maximum degree of pain that a person can tolerate). The most common current pain assessment tool is the 1-10 scale:

- 0 = no pain
- 1-2 = mild pain
- 3-5 = moderate pain
- 6-7 = severe pain
- 8-9 = very severe pain
- 10 = excruciating pain

However, there is more to pain assessment than a number on a scale. Assessment includes information about onset, duration, and intensity. Identifying what triggers pain and what relieves it can be very useful when developing a plan for pain management. Patients may show very different behavior when they are in pain: some may cry and moan with minor pain and others may exhibit little difference in behavior when truly suffering; thus, judging pain by behavior can lead to the wrong conclusions.

Patients with cognitive impairment or inability to verbalize pain
Patients with cognitive impairment or inability to verbalize pain may not be able to indicate the degree of pain, even by using a face scale with pictures of smiling to crying faces. The Pain Assessment in Advanced Dementia (PAINAD) scale may be helpful. Careful observation of non-verbal behavior can indicate that the patient is in pain:

- Respirations: Patients often have more rapid and labored breathing as pain increases with short periods of hyperventilation or Cheyne-Stokes respirations.
- Vocalization: Patients may remain negative in speech or speak quietly and reluctantly. They may moan or groan. As pain increases, they may call out, moan or groan loudly, or cry.
- Facial expression: Patients may appear sad or frightened, may frown or grimace, especially on activities that increase pain.
- Body language: Patients may be tense, fidgeting, pacing and as pain increases may become rigid, clench fists, or lie in fetal position. They may become increasingly combative.
- Consolability: Patients are less distractible or consolable with increased pain.

Consequences of pain

Part of managing pain is understanding patients' perceptions regarding pain and the consequences. Some expect and accept pain and others lack the cognizant awareness to express that they are in pain. Pain, however, is very debilitating and limits quality of life for many patients:
- Limited activity: Patients may be unable to stand, walk, or do their jobs, resulting in their being more sedentary, impairing circulation.
- Frustration: Acute or chronic pain can lead to depression and anger, as well as withdrawal from activities or lack of desire to try new activities. Patients may withdraw from friends and family.
- Additionally, pain has physiological consequences:
- Wound care: Adequate care of the wound may be limited by pain during treatment. Patients may not carry out prescribed treatments or may refuse treatments.
- Perfusion: Pain can result in peripheral vasoconstriction, decreasing perfusion of tissue and impairing leukocyte activity. This, in turn, depresses angiogenesis, further impairing healing of the wound and continuing the cycle of pain.

Considerations regarding pain control measures

Good wound care must include the assessment and management of pain. Dressing changes, especially, are often very painful. There are a number of considerations:
- Pain assessment should be done regularly, allowing the patient to describe the type and extent of pain as well as response to analgesia in order to manage pain optimally.
- Poor perfusion and infection increase pain, so measures should aim at increasing circulation/oxygenation of the wound and assessing for signs of infection and instituting treatment.

- Increasing fluid intake and providing proper nutrition improve wound condition and reduce pain.
- Pain medications should be given as needed and prior to dressing changes. With severe pain, such as burns, patient-controlled analgesia (PCA) devices help the patient feel more independent and relieve fear of pain. Medications to relieve anxiety may potentiate pain medications.
- Fungating cancerous lesions may require modifications in dressing routines to decrease dressing changes and periwound care to prevent painful maceration.

Types of pain

There are two primary types of pain: nociceptive (acute) pain and neuropathic pain although some people may have a combination. Nociceptive or acute pain is the normal nerve response to a painful stimulus. Trauma that results in nociceptive pain can cause severe inflammation and damage to nerve endings. Nociceptive pain usually correlates with extent and type of injury: the greater the injury, the greater the pain. It may be procedural pain (related to wound manipulation and dressing changes) or surgical pain (related to cutting of tissue). It may also be continuous or cyclic, depending upon the type of injury. This type of pain is usually localized to the area of injury and resolves over time as healing takes place. This type of pain is often described as aching or throbbing, but generally responds to analgesia. Uncontrolled, this type of pain can in time result in changes in the nervous system that lead to chronic neuropathic pain.

While nociceptive pain is acute, neuropathic pain is more chronic. Neuropathic pain occurs when there is a primary lesion in the nervous system or dysfunction related to damaged nerve fibers. Neuropathic pain may be associated with conditions such as diabetes, cancer, or traumatic injury to the nervous system. This type of pain is common in chronic wounds and is more often described as burning, stabbing, electric, or shooting pains. Often the underlying pathology causing the pain is not reversible. Pain may be visceral (diffuse or cramping pain of internal organs) caused by injuries to internal organs. It is also often diffuse rather than localized. It may also be somatic pain (involving muscles, skin, bones, and joints). Neuropathic pain is often more difficult to assess that nociceptive pain because the damage may alter normal pain responses. Neuropathic pain often responds better to antidepressants and anti-seizure medications than analgesics.

Pharmacologic treatment of wound pain

Topical anesthetics
There are numerous different types of pain medications that may be used to control pain from wounds, including topical anesthetics:

- Lidocaine 2-4% is frequently used during debridement or dressing changes. Lidocaine is useful only superficially and may take 15-30 minutes before it is effective.
- Eutectic Mixture of Local Anesthetics (EMLA Cream) provides good pain control. The wound is first cleansed and then the cream is applied thickly (1/4 inch) extending about 1/2 inch past the wound to the peri-wound tissue. The wound is then covered with plastic wrap, which is secured and left in place for about 20 minutes. The wrapped time may be extended to 45-60 minute if necessary to completely numb the tissue. The tissue should remain numb for about 1 hour after the plastic wrap is removed, allowing time for the wound to be cleansed, debrided, and/or redressed.

Systemic medications
Systemic medications may be given orally or by injection into muscles, subcutaneous tissue, or veins. The 3-step World Health Organization (WHO) "Analgesic Ladder" is frequently used as a point of reference. Combinations of drugs are often more effective than one alone:

- Step 1: Mild to moderate pain is treated with aspirin, acetaminophen, and NSAIDs.
- Step 2: Moderate to severe pain unrelieved by Step 1 medications may need opioids, such as codeine, tramadol, or Percocet®.
- Step 3: Severe pain without relief from Step 1 or Step 2 medications may need stronger opioids, such as morphine, Dilaudid®, or MS-Contin®.

Note: Meperidine (Demerol®) should not be used for pain control because prolonged use may result in dependence, high doses may cause seizures, and a metabolite of meperidine (normeperidine) may accumulate. It is short acting and peaks quickly but may be indicated for occasional use.

Regional anesthesia
Regional anesthesia (injectable subcutaneous and perineural medications) is used locally about the wound or to provide nerve blocks. Medications include lidocaine, bupivacaine and tetracaine in solution. Epinephrine is sometimes added to increase vasoconstriction and reduce bleeding although it is avoided in distal areas of the limbs (hands and feet) to prevent ischemia. Field blockade involves injecting the anesthetic into the periwound tissue or into the wound margins. The effect may be decreased by inflammation. The effects last for limited periods of time. Regional nerve blocks may involve single injections, the effects of which are limited in duration but can provide pain relief for treatments. Techniques that use continuous catheter infusions are longer lasting and can be controlled more precisely. Blocks

may involve nerves proximal to affected areas, such as peripheral nerve blocks, or large nerve blocks near the spinal cord, such as percutaneous lumbar sympathetic blocks (LSB). Long-term blocks may use alcohol-based medications to permanently inactivate the nerves.

Non-analgesic pain control measures

Non-analgesic pain control measures begin with good communication between the patient and the healthcare provider and an assessment of the causes of pain, which can then be targeted for pain reduction.

- Cleansing of wound: Use normal saline and gentle flushing of wound rather than cytotoxic agents, such as antiseptics, which may cause burning and discomfort.
- Peri-wound care: Use skin sealants to protect intact skin from maceration and skin barriers over denuded skin.
- Wound debridement: Use autolysis when possible.
- Dressings: Select dressings with the goal of reducing pain as well as healing the wound. Moisture-retentive dressings often decrease pain. Avoid wet-to-dry dressings. Decrease frequency of dressing changes if possible.
- Inflammation: Elevate limb if indicated; provide medications to control.
- Edema: Elevate limbs and use compression dressings and sequential compression pumps as indicated.
- Positioning: Use body supports to stabilize wounds when possible. Use turning sheets. Try splinting or immobilizing a wound area.

Nutritional assessment

Initial assessment
Nutritional assessment should be done within the first 24 hours of care to ensure that nutritional requirements are met. The history and physical exam should include the following information about the previous 3 months:

- Changes in food intake, including number of meals eaten daily
- Weight loss (or gain)
- Episodes of depression or stress that may relate to dietary intake
- A sample of a usual daily menu should be developed. Additional screening should include:
  - Daily number of protein, fruit, grain, and vegetable servings
  - Usual fluid intake, including type, amount, and frequency
  - Method of feeding, independent or assisted
  - Mobility
  - Mental status
  - Body Mass Index (BMI), midarm circumference, and calf circumference

- o Living status (independent or dependent)
- o Prescription and non-prescription drugs
- o Pressure sores or other wounds or skin problems

Physical assessment

The physical assessment is an important part of nutritional assessment to determine malnutrition or problems with self-feeding:

- Hair may be dry and brittle or thinning.
- Skin may show poor turgor, ecchymosis, tears, pressure areas, ulcerations, abrasions, or other compromises.
- Mouth may show dry mucous membranes. Lips may have cheilosis, cracking at the corners, and scaly lips (riboflavin deficiency). Gums may be swollen or bleeding, teeth loose or needing care, or dentures poorly fitting. Tongue may be inflamed, dry, cracked, or have sores.
- Nails may become brittle. Spoon shaped or pale nail bed indicates low iron.
- Hands may be crippled or arthritic, making eating difficult.
- Vision may be compromised so that people can't see to prepare food or have difficulty feeding them.
- Mental status may be impaired to the point that people can't understand diet instructions or prepare or eat meals.
- Motor skills may decrease, including hand-mouth coordination or ability to hold utensils.

Nutritional assessment tools

The MNA® (Mini-Nutritional Assessment) by Nestle Nutrition is designed for nutritional assessment of those over age 65 and is only valid for that population. It is a screening and assessment tool to determine the risk for malnutrition and comprises 15 questions about dietary habits and 4 measurements, including Body Mass Index (BMI) using height and weight, mid-arm and calf circumference. The Nutritional Screening Initiative® is another tool for geriatric patients and screens for dietary information as well as social and environmental factors, such as whether the person eats alone, prepares meals, drinks alcohol, and has sufficient income. The Subjective Global Assessment® assesses nutritional status by a thorough history and physical examination. The history assesses weight change, dietary intake, gastro-intestinal symptoms and functional impairment. The results of this assessment tool are evaluated subjectively and scores assigned to determine if malnutrition risks are normal to severe.

Malnutrition

Risk factors and indicators
There are a number of risk factors for malnutrition:
- Hypermetabolism resulting from various diseases, such as AIDS, and trauma, stress, or infection.
- Weight loss, especially sudden or loss of 10% of normal weight over a 3-month period.
- Low body weight of <90% of ideal body weight for age or Low Body Mass Index (BMI) <18.5.
- Immunosuppressive drugs interfere with absorption of nutrients
- Malabsorption of nutrients caused by diseases, such as chronic failure of kidneys or liver.
- Changes in appetite that decrease intake of nutrients.
- Food intolerances, such as lactose intolerance, resulting from lack of enzymes needed to completely digest food so it can be absorbed into the blood stream from the small intestine.
- Dietary restrictions, such as limiting of protein with kidney failure.
- Functional limitations such as inability to feed oneself.
- Lack of teeth or dentures, limiting intake.
- Alterations of taste or smell that render food unpalatable.

Types and symptoms
Protein malnutrition (kwashiorkor or hypoalbuminemia), inadequate protein but adequate fats and carbohydrates, can result from chronic diarrhea, renal disease, infection, hemorrhage, burns, traumatic injuries or other illnesses. Onset is usually rapid with loss of visceral protein while skeletal muscle mass is retained, so it may be difficult to detect on a physical exam. Symptoms include:
- Hypoalbuminemia and anemia
- Edema
- Delayed healing of wound
- Immuno-incompetence

Protein-calorie malnutrition (marasmus), inadequate protein and calories, is usually more obvious. Visceral protein is usually intact as is immune function because weight loss is gradual. However, patients are often very thin or emaciated from loss of skeletal muscle mass. Many are elderly and have chronic illnesses. Symptoms include:
- Decreased basal metabolism
- Lack of subcutaneous fat
- Tissue turgor
- Bradycardia
- Hypothermia

Mixed protein-calorie malnutrition (combination) is common in hospitalized patients and has an acute onset with low visceral protein as well as rapid loss of weight, skeletal muscle mass, and fat.

<u>Starvation and excessive intake</u>
In response wounds, the stress response causes a hypermetabolic state, and caloric and protein needs increase markedly at the same time intake decreases, leading to periods of starvation:
- A short period can result in increased nitrogen in urine and increased output with rapid loss of muscle and weight.
- A prolonged period results in slower weight and muscle loss but can lead to metabolic acidosis with increased ammonia in urine and decreased nitrogen.
- An extended period becomes premorbid with obvious cachexia and weight loss. The midarm muscle circumference decreases and there is increase in creatinine/height index and urinary urea as well as decrease in serum albumin, transferrin and lymphocytes.

Excessive intake may cause obesity, which delays wound healing, but it does not necessarily mean nutrition is adequate. Overweight people can still have inadequate protein, vitamins, and minerals. Because protein and caloric requirements for healing are tied to weight, nutritional needs are high, but fat stores help people to tolerate prolonged periods of starvation.

Dietary changes to add protein

There are a number of dietary changes that can add adequate protein, calories, and needed nutrients to the diet. In some people, co-morbid conditions such as diabetes or high cholesterol should be considered because some foods, such as cheese, are high in sodium and fat, which may be restricted. Increased protein:
- Add meat to vegetarian dishes, such as soups and pastas
- Add milk powder to many foods during preparation
- Substitute milk for water in soups, hot cereals, and cocoa.
- Add cheese to dishes, such as pastas and casseroles.
- Provide high protein drinks, such as High Protein Ensure®.
- Use peanut butter on bread and apples.
- Add extra eggs to dishes, such as custards and meat loaf

Increased calories:
- Use whole milk or cream rather than low fat or non-fat milk
- Add butter, sour cream, or whipping cream to foods.
- Provide frequent snacks.

Nutritional factors that affect skin's ability to remain intact and/or heal

Nutritional status is very important for maintaining the integrity of the skin. People who are on restrictive diets or do not have adequate protein in their diets will lack the amino acids for protein synthesis. A diet too low in fats can be deficient in essential fatty acids, which the skin cells need for the lipid barrier. Carbohydrates are necessary for the cell to carry out basic functions of metabolism. Vitamin A helps to repair skin tissue. Vitamin B complex, especially biotin, is critical form skin formation and prevents dryness and itching. Vitamins C and E have been shown to reduce and counter the negative effects of ultraviolet radiation caused by exposure to the sun. Since Vitamin C is utilized for collagen formation, it is essential that intake is adequate. Minerals, such as iron, selenium, zinc, and copper are important also.

Management of nutritional factors that affect wound healing

Nutritional management must be designed according to individual needs based on many factors, such as age, weight, size, nutritional status, co-morbidity, and size and severity of wound. However, the average healthy person requires about 0.8g of protein per kilogram every day (40-70 g). However, if a person has a wound, then not only must the person have adequate calories and general nutrition but daily added protein and vitamins as well.

- Protein amounts are increased to 1.25 to 2.0 g per kilogram
- Vitamin A 1600-2000 retinal equivalents
- Vitamin C 100-1000 mg
- Zinc 15-30 mg
- B vitamins 200% of RDA
- Iron 20-30 mg

Caloric and fluid intake should be monitored carefully to ensure that the person is eating food that is served. Gastrointestinal tube feedings or parenteral feedings may be necessary if the person cannot take food and fluids orally. Prealbumin levels should be monitored regularly as well.

Wound Etiology and Description

Chronic wounds

Acute wounds heal fairly quickly, moving through stages of healing in a predictable manner; however chronic wounds behave much differently and outcomes are less predictable. There are a number of factors related to chronic wounds:

- Wound nature: chronic wounds are often related to underlying pathology, such as arterial insufficiency, rather than acute injury. Also, the lack of initial bleeding may impair fibrin production and release of growth factors.
- Difference in healing: the initial inflammatory stage of healing is often prolonged because of vascular insufficiency, necrosis, or bacteria.
- Insufficient growth factors: Growth factors are necessary to repair tissue, but there are insufficient numbers or they break down quickly, resulting in cellular senescence (inability of cells to proliferate or respond to growth factors).
- Host factors: Many factors, such as malnutrition and smoking, may interfere with healing.
- Denervation: Lack of adequate innervation impairs the inflammatory response and interferes with healing.

Partial-thickness and full-thickness wounds

Partial-thickness wounds involve only the epidermis and the upper parts of the dermis, so the underlying structures that repair skin and provide nutrients, such as the vasculature, and protection, such as the glands remain intact. Bleeding activates hemostasis and provides a temporary bacterial barrier. Coagulation occurs and fibrin is formed with the clot sealing disrupted vessels. This is followed by fibrinolysis, during which the clot breaks down and repair begins with the inflammatory stage. Healing phase's progress and wounds usually heal within about 2 weeks. Full-thickness wounds involve the loss of the epidermis and dermis and may also involve loss of underlying tissues, through the fascia, muscle, and to the bone. Full-thickness wounds may be acute or chronic and heal by primary or secondary intention. Those healing by secondary intention are usually surgical wounds that have dehisced or those resulting from underlying morbidities that interfere with normal healing. Bleeding and hemostasis do not occur with healing by secondary intention, compromising the healing process.

Classification of wounds

Wounds are classified according to the cause:

- Vascular changes can result in wounds that occur most commonly in the lower extremities, such as those that result from arterial insufficiency and ischemia, those that relate to changes in the lymphatic system, and those related to venous insufficiency.
- Neuropathic changes that occur with chronic diseases, such as diabetes, and chronic alcoholism can decrease sensation and circulation, resulting in ulcerations.
- Shear friction and pressure, especially over bony prominences such as the sacral area and heels, causes erosion of the tissue.
- Trauma often results in contaminated wounds.
- Surgery can involve wounds that are originally contaminated or originally clean, depending upon the type of surgery and the reason.
- Inflammation and infection may result in deteriorating wounds or fistulas.
- Self-inflicted wounds vary widely, from minor cuts to traumatic gunshot wounds.
- Hypergranulation/keloid formation can change the character of a wound and prevent adequate healing.

Pressure ulcers

Assessment

When assessing an ulcer, it is necessary to determine if it is a non-pressure or pressure ulcer because the treatment protocol may vary depending upon whether the ulcer is caused by pressure, venous or arterial insufficiency, or neuropathic disorders. The clinical basis for this determination should be clearly outlined.

- The ulcer should be classified according to the stage and the characteristics, including size (length, width, and depth).
- Pain associated with the ulcer should be described.
- Photographs should be taken if a protocol is in place.
- Ulcers should be monitored daily and any changes carefully documented.
- The ulcer should be evaluated for signs of infection.

It is important to differentiate between colonization, which is very common, and infection, which usually presents with symptoms such as peri-wound erythema and induration and increased pain as well as delayed healing of wound. Wound culture and blood tests should be done if there are indications of infection. Treatment should be determined according to characteristics of the wound.

<u>Causes</u>
Pressure ulcers, also known as decubitus ulcer, are caused primarily by pressure, but there are numerous considerations:

- Pressure intensity: Capillary closing pressure (10-32 Hg) is the minimal pressure needed to collapse capillaries, reducing tissue perfusion. This pressure can be easily exceeded in the sitting or supine position if weight is not shifted.
- Duration of pressure: Low pressure for long periods and high pressure for short periods can both result in pressure ulcers.
- Tissue tolerance: The tissue tolerance is the ability of the skin to tolerate and redistribute pressure, preventing anoxia. Both extrinsic and intrinsic factors can affect tissue tolerance. Extrinsic factors include shear (the skin stays in place but the underlying tissue slides), friction (moving the skin against bedding or other objects), and moisture. Intrinsic factors include poor nutrition, advanced age, low blood pressure, stress, smoking, and low body temperature.

Shear and friction: Shear occurs when the skin stays in place and the underlying tissue in the deep fascia over the bony prominences stretches and slides, damaging vessels and tissue and often resulting in undermining. Shear is one of the most common causes of ulcers, which are often described as pressure ulcers but are technically somewhat different although the effects of shearing are often combined with pressure. The most common cause of shear is elevation of the head of the bed over 30°. Friction against the sheets holds the skin in place while the body slides down the bed, resulting in pressure and damage in the sacrococcygeal area. The underlying vessels are damaged and thrombosed, leading to undermining and deep ulceration. Friction is a significant cause of pressure ulcers because it acts with gravity to cause shear. Friction by itself results only in damage to the epidermis and dermis, such as abrasions or denudement referred to as "sheet burn." Friction and pressure can combine, however, to form ulcers.

<u>Staging system</u>
The National Pressure Ulcer Advisory Panel developed a staging system to ensure that definitions for pressure ulcers were standardized.

- Stage I: Nonblanchable erythema – Intact, reddened area that does not blanch (Difficult to assess in darker skin). Area remains intact but the physical appearance is altered.
- Stage II: Partial thickness – Destruction of the epidermis and/or dermis. This type of injury may be an intact blister, ruptured blister, or an open ulcer if it has a pinkish or a reddish wound bed.
- Stage III: Full thickness skin loss – Epidermis and dermis have experienced loss and the injury now extends through to the subcutaneous fat tissue. Tunneling could be present. Muscle, tendons, and bones have not been injured.

- Stage IV: Full thickness tissue loss – Damage has progressed to bone, muscle, or tendons. There is often tunneling present, osteomyelitis is common, and the depth of the ulcer will vary by location.
- Unstageable/Unclassified – Injury is present and involves full thickness, but cannot be staged until slough is removed.
- Suspected Deep Tissue Injury – Discolored skin that is still intact but has been damaged. Suspect it is deeper than stage I, but the epidermis is still intact

At risk populations
Populations at risk for pressure ulcers include the following;
- The elderly, especially those with impairment of mobility or changes to the skin experience the most pressure ulcers, often associated with hospitalization or long term care. For those admitted to long term care facilities, 10-18% have at least one ulcer on admission.
- People with spinal cord injuries are at risk because of loss of sensation. About 20-30% have spinal cord injuries, but up to 85% will develop a pressure ulcer at some time.
- Children who are hospitalized are also at risk, but rates vary widely depending upon the child's condition and the setting. Rates in pediatric care units may be as high as 27% and 20% in neonatal intensive care units. Ulcers usually occur within the first 2 days after admission.
- Surgical patients have pressure ulcer rates of 4-45%, depending on age, nutrition, and co-morbidities. Tissue damage may not be evident for up to 3 days after injury.

Arterial and venous insufficiency

There are multiple characteristics that distinguish arterial from venous insufficiency:
- Type of pain:
  - Arterial: ranges from intermittent claudication to severe constant.
  - Venous: aching and cramping.
- Pulses:
  - Arterial: weak or absent
  - Venous: present
- Skin of extremity:
  - Arterial: rubor on dependency but pallor of foot on elevation. Skin is pale, shiny, and cool with loss of hair on toes and foot. Nails are thick and ridged.
  - Venous: brownish discoloration around ankles and anterior tibial area.

- Characteristics of ulcers:
  - o Arterial: Painful, deep, circular, often necrotic ulcers on toe tips, toe webs, heels or other pressure areas with little edema of extremity.
  - o Venous: Varying degrees of pain in superficial, irregular ulcers on medial or lateral malleolus and sometimes anterior tibial area with moderate to severe edema of extremity.

Diabetic foot ulcers

Most diabetic ulcers are on the foot, ranging from the toes to the heels. Ulcers may first appear as laceration, blisters, or punctures, and the wound is usually circular with well-defined edges. There is often callus in the periwound tissue.
Common sites:
- Toes: The toes are frequent sites for ulcers because of the potential for trauma. The interphalangeal joints often have limited flexibility that causes pressure and friction. The dorsal toes may have hammertoes from injuries or improperly fitted shoes that are easily injured. Distal toes may suffer injury from poor perfusion, heat, or short footwear.
- Metatarsal heads may have poor flexibility, increasing pressure.
- Bunions may erode because of deformities or narrow footwear.
- Midfoot may suffer injury from trauma or Charcot's fracture.
- Heels are susceptible to unrelieved pressure, often related to prolonged periods of bed rest.

SAD classification system for lower-extremity neuropathic disease

The Size, Area, Depth (SAD) classification system for lower-extremity neuropathic disease is one of many that builds upon the original or modified Wagner classification system and assigns a 0-3 grade based on 5 categories: area, depth, sepsis, arteriopathy, and denervation.
- 0. No pathology evident.
- 1. Ulcer is <10mm^2, involving subcutaneous tissue with superficial slough or exudate, diminution or absence of pulses, and reduced sensation.
- 2. Ulcer is 10-20 mm^2, extending to tendon, joint, capsule, or periosteum with cellulitis, absence of pulses except for neuropathy dominant ulcers that have palpable pedal pulses.
- 3. Ulcer is >30 mm^2, extending to bones and/or joints, with osteomyelitis, gangrene, and Charcot's foot.

This, as most other classification systems, is useful but doesn't distinguish between those wounds that follow an atypical pattern or may be consistent with the grade in some areas and inconsistent in others.

Modified Wagner Ulcer Classification System

The modified Wagner Ulcer Classification System divides foot ulcers into six grades, based on lesion depth, osteomyelitis or gangrene, infection, ischemia, and neuropathy:

- 0. At risk but no open ulcers.
- 1. Superficial ulcer, extending into subcutaneous tissue; superficial infection with or without cellulitis.
- 2. Full-thickness ulcer to tendon or joint with no abscess or osteomyelitis.
- 3. Full-thickness ulcer that may extend to bone with abscess, osteomyelitis, or sepsis of joint and may include deep plantar infections, abscesses, fascitis, or infections of tendon sheath.
- 4. Gangrene of area of foot but the rest of foot is salvageable.
- 5. Gangrene of entire foot, requiring amputation.

While this classification system is useful in predicting outcomes, it does not contain information about the size of the ulcer or the type of infection, so it should be only one part of an assessment, as more detailed information is needed to fully evaluate an ulcer.

Arterial, venous, and neuropathic ulcers

Locations:
- Arterial: Ends of toes pressure points, traumatic nonhealing wounds.
- Neuropathic: Plantar surface, metatarsal heads, toes and sides of feet.
- Venous: Between knees and ankles, medial malleolus.

Wound bed characteristics:
- Arterial: Pale, necrotic.
- Neuropathic: Red (or ischemic).
- Venous: Dark red, fibrinous slough.

Types of exudate:
- Arterial: Slight amount, infection common.
- Neuropathic: Moderate to large amounts, infection common.
- Venous: Moderate to large amounts.

Wound perimeters:
- Arterial: Circular, well-defined
- Neuropathic: Circular, well defined and often with callous formation.
- Venous: Irregular, poorly defined.

Pain:
- Arterial: Very painful.
- Neuropathic: Often absent because of reduced sensation.
- Venous: Pain varies.

Skin:
- Arterial: Pale, friable, shiny, and hairless, with dependent rubor and elevational pallor.

- Neuropathic: Ischemic signs (as in arterial) may be evident with co-morbidity.
- Venous: Brownish discoloration of ankles and shin, edema common.

Elements of wound assessment

Wound margins
Wound margins and the tissue surrounding the wound should be described carefully and with correct terminology:
- Color should be described using color descriptions and such terms as blanched, erythematous (red), or ecchymosed (purple, green, yellow).
- Skin texture may be normal, indurated (hardened), or edematous (swollen). Note if there is cellulitis or maceration evident.
- Wound edges may be diffuse (without clear margins), well defined, or rolled. A healing ridge may be evident if granulation has begun. Note if the wound is closed (as with a surgical incision) or open (as with dehiscence or ulcerations). Note if wound edges are attached or unattached (indicating undermining or tunneling).
- Tunneling or undermining should be assessed by probing the wound margins with a moist sterile cotton applicator, using clock face locators (toward the head is 12 o'clock, for example). Tunneling may be described as extending from 3 o'clock to 4 o'clock. A large area is usually described as undermining. The size should be measured or estimated as closely as possible.

Distribution, drainage, and odor
Distribution of lesions should be clearly delineated if there is more than one lesion over an area. The arrangement of the lesions can be helpful for diagnosis and treatments.
- Linear (in a line)
- Satellites (small lesions around a larger one)
- Diffuse (scattered freely over an area)

Drainage may vary considerably from nothing at all to copious outpourings of discharge.
- Serous drainage is usually clear to slightly yellow.
- Serosanguineous drainage is a combination of serous drainage and blood.
- Sanguineous drainage is bloody.
- Purulent discharge may be thick and milky, yellow, brownish, or green, depending upon the infective agent

Odor requires more subjective assessment, but the odor and type of discharge together can provide useful information. Some infective agents, such as *Pseudomonas,* produce distinctive odors, which may be described in various ways: Musty/Foul/Sweet.

Location and size
Wound location should be described in terms of anatomic position using landmarks (such as sternal notch, umbilicus, lateral malleolus), correct medical terminology, and directional terms:
- Anterior (in front)
- Posterior (behind)
- Superior (above)
- Inferior (below)

Wound size should be carefully described through actual measurement rather than association (the size of a dime). Measurements should be done with a disposable ruler in millimeters or centimeters. The current standard for measurement:

Length X width X depth = dimension

However, a clear description requires more detail. The measurement should be done at the greatest width and greatest length. More than 2 measurements may be needed if the wound is very irregularly shaped. The depth of the wound should be measured by inserting a sterile applicator and grasping or marking the applicator at skin level and then measuring the length below. Ideally, the wound should be photographed as well following protocols for photography.

Wound bed tissue
Distribution of lesions should be clearly delineated if there is more than one lesion over an area. The arrangement of the lesions can be helpful for diagnosis and treatments.
- Linear (in a line)
- Satellites (small lesions around a larger one)
- Diffuse (scattered freely over an area)

Wound bed tissue should be described as completely as possible, including color and general appearance:
- Granulation tissue should be slightly granular in appearance and deep pink to bright red and moist, bleeding easily if disturbed.
- Clean non-granular tissue is smooth and deep pink or red and is not healing.
- Hypergranulation is excessive soft flaccid granulating tissue that is raised above the level of the periwound tissue, preventing proper epithelization, and may reflect excess moisture in the wound,
- Epithelization should appear at wound edges first and then eventually cover the wound. It is dry and light pink or violet in color.
- Slough is necrotic tissue that is viscous, soft and yellow-gray in appearance and adheres to the wound.
- Eschar is hard dark brown or black leathery necrotic tissue that accumulates with death of the tissue.

- 48 -

Wound infection

<u>Assessment</u>

There are a number of different aspects to assessment for wound infection:

- Patient history: A complete history is critical. Any prior hospitalizations or recent surgeries should be noted as well as medication history. The history should show when and how the wound first occurred to help determine if the wound is acute or chronic. Co-morbidities should be noted as well as age and cognitive, functional, and nutritional status.
- Examination: A complete assessment of the wound, noting wound characteristics and drainage, should be done along with a careful and complete physical examination.
- Laboratory testing: Laboratory findings provide indications of the type and extent of infection and should include the complete blood count to determine if there is elevation of the white blood count. Wound cultures and sensitivities should be done to identify the microorganism and treatment. CT scans may be done to identify abscesses.

<u>Stages</u>

The skin contains natural flora that cause no problem with intact skin, but if the skin barrier is breached, these microorganisms can migrate in to an open wound. Additionally, some pathogens, such as *Staphylococcus aureus,* are endemic to hospital environments and can contaminate wounds. There is a continuum to the infectious process:

- Colonization occurs when microorganism replicate. There may be superficial signs of infection, but this phase is not pathogenic and should not be treated with antibiotics.
- Critical colonization occurs when the bioburden increases, arresting healing of the wound. Wounds may appear red and clean but lack granulation. The infection remains localized, and there is no systemic response. Topical antibiotics may be used at this phase.
- Infection occurs when the microorganisms invade the tissue and there is a systemic response. Acute wounds show signs of inflammation, but chronic wounds may only exhibit increased pain, exudate, or further delay in healing. Cultures and sensitivities should be done to ascertain the correct treatment.

Complications of wounds

Complications of wounds include:

- Hemorrhage: Macerated tissue becomes soft and weakened, increasing risk of trauma and hemorrhage, which may occur as tissue and blood vessels erode. Subcutaneous bleeding or hemorrhage is usually indicated by purple ecchymosis. In some cases, frank bleeding or oozing may occur and/or a hematoma may form.

- Dehiscence: The incision becomes disrupted because of infection, inadequate suturing, suture rejection, or stress (such as from coughing). The wound edges usually begin to slowly separate, and serosanguineous and/or purulent (with infection) drainage is usually evident. The wound is most at risk for dehiscence in the first 14 days. Often dehiscence is mild because of a suture or staple coming lose, but if the entire wound opens, this is a medical emergency.
- Evisceration: After the wound dehisces, the wound contents begin to protrude through the opening. This is especially critical with abdominal wounds because the intestines may suddenly erupt through the opening. Patients often feel as though something is "giving way" and may feel pain and nausea. This is always a medical emergency.

Surgical site infections

<u>CDC classification</u>
The CDC classifies surgical site infections as superficial incisional, deep incisional, or organ/space, depending on the severity of the infection.
- Superficial incisional:
  - Occurs within 30 days of surgery
  - Purulent discharge evident, organisms isolated, signs of infection and wound opened by surgeon, or diagnosis by physician.
- Deep incisional:
  - Occurs within 30 days of surgery if no implant or 1 year if implant in place.
  - Purulent discharge evident, signs of infections and incision dehisces or is deliberately opened by physician.
  - Abscess or other evidence of infection found on examination, radiology, or histopathology.
  - Diagnosis by physician.
- Organ space:
  - Occurs within 30 days of surgery is no implant or 1 year if implant in place if infection appears related.
  - Infection involves any part of body (organs, tissues) manipulated during surgery.
  - Purulent discharge evident from drain to organ/space, organisms isolated from fluids or tissue in organ space, abscess in area, or diagnosis by physician

<u>Risk factors</u>
Risk factors should be carefully assessed to determine the likelihood of surgical site infections:

- Duration of surgery: Surgeries more than 2 hours in length increase risk.
- Co-morbidity: Some conditions, such as diabetes mellitus or skin disease in surgical area, predispose patients to infection.
- Steroids: Immunosuppressive response allows infection.
- Malnutrition: Nutrients needed for healing are lacking.
- Recent surgery: Each procedure increases risk.
- Extended hospitalization: Risk increases with length of hospitalization prior to surgery.
- Staphylococcus aureus: Nasal colonization or presence on skin allows bacteria to migrate to wound.
- Remote infection: Infection anywhere else in the body poses risk.
- Prior radiation: Radiation therapy compromises tissue and delays healing, allowing for infection to occur more easily.
- Old/young: The very young and elderly are more easily infected.
- Circulatory impairment: Hypoxemia or localized impairment, such as with peripheral vascular disease, compromise tissue. Smoking interferes with circulation as well.

Surgical/vascular interventions for arterial insufficiency/ ulcers

The goals of management for arterial insufficiency and ulcers are to improve perfusion and save the limb, but lifestyle changes and medications may be insufficient.   There are a number of indications for surgical intervention:

- Poor healing prognosis includes those with ABI < 0.5 because their perfusion is severely compromised.
- Failure to respond to conservative treatment (medications and lifestyle changes) even with an ABI > 0.5.
- Intolerable pain, such as with severe intermittent claudication, which is incapacitating and limits the patient's ability to work or carry out activities. Rest pain is an indication that medical treatment is insufficient.
- Limb-threatening condition, such as severe ischemia with increasing pain at rest, infection, and/or gangrene. Infection can cause a wound to deteriorate rapidly.

Surgical intervention is indicated only for those patients with patent distal vessels as demonstrated by radiologic imaging procedures.

Surgical/ vascular interventions for treatment of severe arterial insufficiency include 3 different types of procedures:

- Bypass grafts in which a section of the saphenous vein or an upper extremity vein are harvested to use to bypass damaged arteries and supply blood to distal vessels. Because veins have valves, they must be reversed or stripped of valves prior to attachment. Synthetic grafts are also sometimes used, but they have a much higher failure rate.

- Angioplasty can be used if disease is not extensive (>10 in length), but arteries must be large enough to accommodate the procedure safely. Initial results are good but long-term rates have been less positive although the use of anticoagulants improves success rates.
- Amputation is the procedure that treatment tries to avoid, but it is sometimes required if ischemia is irreversible or if there is severe necrosis and infection that is life threatening.

Excessive scarring

Excessive scarring includes hypertrophic and keloid scars, which are characterized by raised scars that are erythematous and itchy. Excessive scarring is more common in darkly pigmented skin or in areas where the tissue may stretch, such as over joints. Young or pregnant patients or those with a family history of excessive scarring are at increased risk. There are some distinctions between hypertrophic and keloid scars:

- Hypertrophic scars most frequently occur over joints where there is tension on the wound. They remain localized to the area of the original wound and may spontaneously regress. They may result in contracture of the wound
- Keloid scars most frequently occur on the upper back and chest as well as the deltoids and earlobes. They extend beyond the original wound and rarely regress. They usually arise after the wound has healed as raised, shiny, rope-like fibrous scars. They do not result in contracture of the wound.

Scarless healing

Scarless healing occurs in the early-gestation fetus, during the first 2 trimesters, but this ability to heal without scars is lost during the 3rd trimester. This is important for intrauterine surgical procedures, commonly performed during the second trimester when abnormalities become evident. The fetus heals without scarring for a variety of reasons:

- Platelet aggregation is lessoned, resulting in less growth factor, such as PDGF.
- The inflammatory response is lessoned because of immaturity of the immune system and lack of inflammatory cytokines.
- Wounds move quickly from the inflammatory to the proliferative stage of healing. Fibroblasts, keratinocytes, and endothelial cells, critical to tissue formation, rapidly cover the wound bed. There is no contraction or scarring of the wound.
- Growth factors are balanced so they stimulate growth of connective tissue but prevent excess from forming.
- New and native collagen is indistinguishable, so the new tissue remains flexible.

Treatment Administration and Management

Wound cleansers

Wound cleansers include:
- Normal saline or sterile water: These are the most commonly used cleansers for wound that are relatively clean with little residue. They may also be used to irrigate wounds that are contaminated with dirt or debris in order to loosen and remove it.
- Skin wash with surfactant: This may be used after irrigation with NS/water if the wound contains residue, slough, or dry, scaly tissue although care must be used to avoid any granulation tissue.
- Antimicrobial skin cleansers: These include alcohol and povidone iodine and are usually reserved for intact skin, as there appears to be no lasting benefit to use on open wounds—although some antimicrobial skin cleansers may be indicated for severely contaminated acute wounds for the initial cleansing.
- Soaps: Most soaps should be avoided because they tend to be alkaline and the pH level of the wound should be maintained at 5 to 6.

Cleansing procedures, solutions, and measures

Cleansing methods should remove surface bacteria, but cleansing must be done carefully to prevent damage to tissue. Wounds should be cleansed at each dressing change. Exudate may be removed carefully with soft gauze or swabs by wiping from the center outward, using a new piece of gauze or swab for each wipe. The wound should then be irrigated to mechanically remove exudate or debris. Irrigation under pressure has been found to cleanse wounds effectively while reducing trauma and infection.
- Optimum pressure is between 8-12 psi
- <4 psi is inadequate
- >15 psi can cause trauma or force bacteria into tissue.

Low-pressure irrigation with 250 ml squeeze bottle delivers 4.5 psi while a 60 ml piston irrigation syringe delivers 4.2 psi. High-pressure irrigation (8-12 psi) utilizing a 35cc syringe with an 18-19 gauge angiocath provides good cleansing. Irrigation solution should be sterile normal saline instead of antimicrobial/antibacterial solutions, which are cytotoxic and may delay healing.

Topical agents for peri-wound skin protection

Skin sealants
While a warm, moist environment is optimum for wound healing, the exudate poses a risk to adjacent tissue, which must be protected or it will macerate and may

ulcerate and increase the size of the wound. Various topical agents are used to protect peri-wound skin, including skin sealants, which are film-forming barriers composed of a polymer in a fast-drying solvent, applied every 1-4 days, depending on the product. When the sealant is applied to the skin, the solvent (often isopropyl alcohol) dissolves, leaving the transparent plasticized polymer barrier over the tissue. It may be applied to intact or irritated tissue although there may be some discomfort from the alcohol solvent with broken skin.

Sealants can be used to protect skin from exudate, urine, stool, chemicals, and adhesive stripping.   Sealants are applied with wipes, wands, or sprays. Some sealant products include:
- Skin Prep®
- Shield Skin®
- Bard® Protective Barrier Film Wipe
- Allkare® Convatec
- Cavilon®No Sting Barrier Film (does not use alcohol).

Moisture barrier paste
Moisture barrier pastes are ointments with powder added to improve absorption and make them more durable and solid, providing a thick skin barrier. Many are zinc oxide based, making them somewhat difficult to remove. Mineral oil is often used to remove the paste. Some paste products now on the market are transparent so that skin can be monitored.   Additionally, some pastes contain karaya or carboxymethyl cellulose to increase adherence to the tissue.   Pastes are frequently used over denuded or excoriated tissue to absorb exudate and protect from drainage, urine, or feces, so they are used for both peri-anal and peri-wound tissues. While pastes are more resistant to drainage than ointments and adhere better to denuded skin, they do interfere with adhesion of dressings, and zinc oxide cannot be used with some wound care treatments. Pastes are usually reapplied with each dressing change without being completely removed first. Some barrier pastes include:
- Critic-Aid® Skin paste
- Ilex® Skin Protectant Paste
- Remedy Calazime® Protectant Paste.

Moisture barrier ointment
Moisture barrier ointments provide protection for the skin from moisture, exudate, urine, and feces with petrolatum or zinc oxide based-products packaged in tubes or small individual packets. These products, because of their greasy nature, can interfere with adhesion of the wound dressings, and some wound care products cannot be used with zinc oxide, so they have limited application. This type of barrier is frequently used with patients who are incontinent to prevent incontinence dermatitis, which can deteriorate into pressure ulcers. Barrier ointments are usually reapplied with each dressing or diaper change, so overall costs may be higher than with barrier films that can be applied less frequently. Some products

contain karaya or carboxymethyl cellulose (hydrophilics) to improve adherence to the skin. Some barrier ointment products include:
- Caloseptine® Ointment
- Lantiseptic ® Skin Protectant
- Proshield Plus® Skin Protectant
- Critic-Aid® Clear Hydrophilic Ointment

Skin barrier powders
Skin barrier powders are used as an initial barrier on denuded skin to provide an adherent base for ointments, pastes, or solid skin adhesive barriers. The powder is sprinkled over the denuded area and excess removed before application of second barrier. They should be applied thinly because excess will impair adhesion of other barrier products, and they should not be used on intact skin, as they will not properly adhere. Skin barrier powders contain powder pectin, karaya, gelatine, carboxymethyl cellulose or combinations. They are frequently used with ostomy products when the skin has become weepy. Warm moist areas are ideal for fungus growth, causing burning and itching, so the addition of antifungal powder may be necessary as well to promote healing. Use of the skin barrier powders should be discontinued as soon as the skin heals. Skin barrier powders include:
- Stomahesive® Protective Powder
- Karaya® Powder
- Premium® Powder

Solid skin barriers
Solid skin barriers are solid waterproof moldable adhesive skin barriers, usually in the form of rings, strips, or wafers that provide skin protection for moisture, exudate, urine, or feces. They may contain hydrocolloids, pectin, karaya, gelatine, carboxymethyl cellulose or combinations. They are frequently used with urostomies and ileostomies as a base to anchor appliances and protect the skin from discharge. They may be cut to fit about snugly about wounds. While they are frequently left in place for days at a time, it is possible for drainage to leak under the barrier, so they must be checked. Some swell when in contact with discharge and have acidic pH to discourage growth of organisms. Solid skin barriers are more durable than ointments or pastes, but they must be removed carefully to prevent stripping of the skin, especially if they are applied in an area that receives pressure, such as the coccyx. Solid skin barriers include:
- Hollister Flextend®
- Stomahesive®
- Eakin®
- Premium® Skin Barrier

Basic requirements for dressings

The basic requirements of dressings, regardless of the type, are the following:
- Maintain a moist environment in order to promote healing.
- Absorb wound drainage and preventing leakage.
- Increase wound temperature to promote healing.
- Provide a protective barrier to prevent mechanical injury to the wound.
- Provide a protective barrier to prevent colonization and infection with microorganisms.
- Allow exchange of gases and fluids.
- Retain and absorb odor of wound or drainage.
- Remove easily without causing additional trauma to the wound or disrupting the healing process.
- Debride wound of dead tissue and exudate.
- Provide protection without toxicity or causing sensitivity reactions.
- Provide a sterile protective covering for the wound.

The dressing that directly covers the wound may be inadequate to absorb large amounts of drainage, so sometimes additional secondary dressings are needed.

Keeping a healing wound warm and moist

One of the basic principles of current wound care is the use of occlusive dressings that keep the wound warm and moist. There are a number of reasons for keeping a healing wound warm and moist:
- Reduction in dehydration allows cells such as neutrophils and fibroblasts to carry out their functions in wound repair, as they require a moist environment. This also results in less cell death.
- Angiogenesis requires a moist environment and low oxygen tension, which is found in occlusive dressings.
- Autolytic debridement with proteolytic enzymes is enhanced in a moist environment.
- Re-epithelization of tissue occurs because the epidermal cells are able to spread across the surface of the wound.
- Reduction in microorganisms because of the seal provided by occlusive dressings decreases infection.
- Pain reduction results from protection of the nerve endings and the need for fewer dressing changes.

Gauze dressings

Gauze dressings are made from cotton, rayon, or polyester, are frequently used with primary closure where there is little or no exudate and the purpose is to provide protection of the partial or full-thickness wounds or those with cavities or tracts. They may be sterile or non-sterile. In the past they were used for wet to dry

- 56 -

dressings, but wet to dry dressings have little use in current wound care unless the wound is very small because the gauze adheres to the wound and can disrupt granulation or epithelization. Wet to moist saline gauze dressings are sometimes used to treat wounds but are less effective than hydrocolloid dressings. Gauze dressings may be used as secondary dressings with another type of dressing in direct contact with the wound or as packing to fill dead space in combination with amorphous hydrogel or other dressings. When used to fill space, the gauze should be fluffed to avoid causing excess pressure.

Choice of dressing

There are a wide variety of dressing products, and there is not one dressing that can suffice for all wounds. Dressings should be chosen according to the type of wound and the function of the dressing. A series of different types of dressings may be used during the healing process. There are 3 main types of dressings to consider when determining which will be the most effective for a particular type of wound:
- Traditional topical dressings that are used primarily to cover the wound, such as gauze and tulle.
- Interactive dressings, such as polymeric films, are generally transparent so that the wound can be observed and are permeable to water vapor and oxygen but provide an effective barrier for microorganisms, such as hyaluronic acid, hydrogels and foam dressings.
- Bioactive dressings provide substances that directly promote wound healing, such as hydrocolloids, alginates, collagens, and chitosan.

Semi-permeable film

Semi-permeable film (OpSite®, Tegaderm®, Polyskin II®) dressings are composed of polyurethane with a coating of acrylic adhesive so the dressing will adhere to the skin. These types of dressings are frequently used over intravenous sites to allow observation of tissue. They are suitable only for shallow partial-thickness wounds that have little or no exudate because they are not able to absorb; therefore, they are not suitable for infected wounds. They are permeable to air and water vapor but provide a barrier to pathogenic agents and liquid. The tissue under the dressing is maintained in a warm moist environment, encouraging autolysis. The dressings are comfortable and may be left in place for up to 1 week although some people may develop local irritation from the adhesive. Semi-permeable film may be used as a protective dressing and is often used for stage I and II pressure ulcers.

Tulle or impregnated gauze dressings

Tulle dressings, also known as paraffin gauze, (Jelonet®, Paranet®) are open weave gauze that are coated with paraffin so they do not adhere to the wound, but are suitable only for flat or shallow wounds. They may be useful for people with

Copyright © Mometrix Media. You have been licensed one copy of this document for personal use only. Any other reproduction or redistribution is strictly prohibited. All rights reserved.

sensitive skin. When these are placed in contact with the wound, secondary dressings may be used to absorb exudate.

Impregnated gauze may contain antimicrobials, medications, nutrients, and moisture (such as normal saline). Commonly used gauzes are impregnated with petrolatum, zinc oxide, and iodoform. They are used for partial or full-thickness wounds or those infected or with cavities or tracts. The choice of gauze depends upon the needs of the wound. They should be loosely packed into cavities and avoid contact with intact skin as they may cause maceration because of the moisture content of the dressing. Exudate should be carefully monitored so dressings can be changed as needed.

Alginates or other fiber gelling dressings

Alginates (AlgiSite M®, Sorbsan®, Aquacel®, Hydrofiber®) are very absorbent dressings made from brown seaweed. Through ion exchange, they absorb drainage and form a hydrophilic gel that conforms to the size and shape of the wound, so they are useful for full-thickness wounds with moderate to heavy exudate or slough, such as pressure ulcers and cavity wounds, especially if there is undermining or tunneling. They are effective for infected and foul-smelling wounds. Alginates are sold in sheet form or fibers for packing. Alginate dressings or packing fibers are loosely packed into the wound to allow for swelling and then secured with a secondary dressing. They are usually changed once daily. Alginates serve to cushion and protect the wound as well as contain exudate. They are easier to remove than gauze dressings used for packing and cause less discomfort. Alginates need differing times to gel with some requiring 24 hours, so they are not interchangeable.

Hydrocolloid dressings

Hydrocolloids (DuoDerm®, Restore®, Tegasorb®) are sheets or wafers of absorbent adherent material with an occlusive coating so that they provide a barrier to moisture. They are used for clean granulating wounds that are partial and full thickness with minimal to moderate amounts of drainage. They may be used with pastes or alginates. Hydrocolloids come in various sizes and shapes and can be cut to fit, overlapping the wound by 2-3 cm. They are usually changed about every 2-5 days. Hydrocolloid material may be stiff and should be warmed between the hands to soften before application. Some hydrocolloids emit an unpleasant odor when active. Because the dressings are occlusive, infected wounds should be observed carefully for signs of infection with anaerobic bacteria. They may be used with compression for venous ulcers but are not recommended for third degree burns. Hydrocolloids may cause hypergranulation tissue to form.

Contact layer dressings

Contact layers (Dermanet®, Mepitel®, Tegapore®) are composed of woven polyamide net and may be coated with silicone (Mepitel®). They adhere lightly to the wound but have pores that allow exudate to pass through to absorbent secondary dressings. They are particularly useful in wounds in which adherence of dressings to the tissue may pose problems, such as with abrasions, second degree burns, grafts, full-thickness granular wounds, and skin damaged by radiotherapy or steroids. They may be used with negative pressure wound therapy. They protect the wound base but are not recommended for shallow or dry wounds. Usually the contact layer stays in place for up to a week while the secondary absorbent dressings are changed more often. If exudate is extremely viscous, it may not penetrate the net and can build up beneath the contact layer. Some types of contact layers may need to be kept moistened with normal saline so they don't adhere to the wound base.

Composite dressings

Composites are combination dressings that are frequently used to secure primary dressings or with other dressings, such as alginates. The material in composites varies from one dressing to another, but usually consists of some type of impermeable exterior barrier to prevent leakage of exudate, an absorptive layer (*not* alginate, foam, hydrocolloid or hydrogel), a semi-adherent or non-adherent surface for covering the wound, and an adhesive rim to secure the dressing to the periwound tissue. Used alone, they are most suitable for partial or shallow full-thickness wounds but used with other dressings they are suitable for larger wounds with minimal to large amounts of exudate. A paper backing must be removed prior to application. They are usually changed about 3 times a week or more often if needed for wounds with larges amount of exudate.

Hydrogel dressings

Hydrogel dressings (AquaForm®, Curasol®, Hypergel®, Elastogel®, Vigilon®, Intrasite® gel) are produced in amorphous form, supplied in tubes, or impregnated in packing strip materials. They are also produced in sheet form, with or without adhesive border. They have a high moisture content with water or glycerin with hydrophilic sites allowing them to absorb exudate and provide a warm, moist wound environment. Hydrogels are used for partial and full-thickness wounds, dry to small amounts of exudate, necrotic and infected wounds. They are applied directly to the wound and provide rehydration and autolysis, effectively and quickly debriding the wound. They are usually used with a secondary dressing, such as gauze or films. Dressings may be changed every 1-3 days, depending upon the type of product used. Hydrogels are contraindicated for wounds with heavy exudate as the leakage may cause maceration of periwound tissue or candidiasis.

Foam/foam film dressings

Foam/foam film dressings are made of semi-permeable hydrophilic foam and sheet forms may have an impermeable barrier. They come in a wide variety of sizes and shapes (wafers, rolls, pillows, films) depending upon the manufacturer. Some types have a charcoal layer to control odor. Foam dressings provide a warm, moist environment and provide cushioning. Foam dressings may be used for partial and full-thickness wounds. Non-sheet forms are used as packing and are appropriate for minimal to heavy exudate. When used as packing, a secondary non-occlusive dressing is secured over the foam. They are used for leg ulcers as well as pressure sores. Because they are intended for wounds with exudate in order to provide the appropriate environment for healing, they are not suitable for dry epithelializing wounds or those with eschar. Sheet forms can be used as secondary dressings with alginates, pastes, or powders. Some have adhesive borders. Foam dressings are changed every 2-7 days, depending on the dressing type and the wound.

Wound pouches

Wound pouches (Convatec® Wound Manager, Hollister® Wound Manager) are adapted from ostomy appliances and work in a similar way to contain heavy exudate from fistulas, wounds, drains, and tubes. The pouches provide a skin barrier to protect the skin and a drainage spout so that the pouch can be attached to straight drainage and a bedside bag. The pouch provides odor control as well. The opening in the pouch is cut to fit around the wound and paste, such as Stomahesive®, is applied about the cut opening to ensure seal. The skin is usually wiped with a skin barrier prior to application, and any skin crevices are filled with paste. Forceps are used to feed drains or tubes through the opening of the pouch. Pouches are usually changed about every 4-7 days or when there is leakage or drainage under appliance.

Absorptive dressings and wound fillers

Absorptive dressings (Surgipad®, Tendersorb®, ABD® pad, Exu-dry®) are composed of cellulose, cotton, or rayon fibers. Some have adhesive borders. They are highly absorptive and are intended for wounds that have moderate to heavy drainage. They are changed every 1-2 days. Wound fillers (Biafine WDE®, DuoDerm® Sterile Hydroactive Paste, Multidex® Maltodextrin Wound Dressing) are composed of starch copolymers in numerous different forms, such as pastes, granules, beads, gels, and powders. They fill dead space in shallow wounds, hydrate, providing a warm moist environment, and absorb exudate. They soften necrotic tissue and aid debridement. Wound fillers are indicated for partial and shallow full-thickness wounds with minimal to moderate exudate and can be used for both infected wounds and uninfected wounds. They are used with secondary dressings, such as films and hydrocolloids. Wound fillers are not recommended for use in dry, eschar-covered, or tunneled wounds. Dressings are usually changed daily.

Topical agents to reduce bacterial load

Topical antibiotics may be used to treat localized wound infections based on results of culture and sensitivities so that the treatment is appropriate for the invading microorganism. Topical antibiotics include:

- Cadexomer Lodine (Iodosorb®) is an iodine preparation formulated to be less toxic to granulating tissue. It is applied as powder, paste, or ointment. The ointment contains beads with iodine. The beads swell in contact with exudate, slowly releasing the iodine, which and is affective against a broad range of bacteria, *Staphylococcus aureus, MRSA, Streptococcus, and Pseudomonas,* as well as viruses and fungi.
- Gentamicin sulphate, prepared as a cream or ointment, is a broad-spectrum antibiotic that is effective against both primary and secondary skin infections in stasis and other ulcers or skin lesions. It is bacteriocidal against *Staphylococcus aureus, Streptococcus, and Pseudomonas,* but does not have antiviral or antifungal properties.
- Metroidazole, prepared as a gel or a wax-glycerin cream, is effective against MRSA infections.
- Mupirocin 2%, prepared in an ointment, is effective primarily against Gram-positive bacteria and is used primarily for *Staphylococcus, MRSA,* and *Streptococcus.* It is frequently used to treat nasal colonization of *Staphylococcus* because colonization is implicated in subsequent wound infections.
- Polymyxin B sulphate-Bacitracin zinc-neomycin ointment (Neosporin®) is frequently used in to prevent infections in small cuts and lacerations, but it can also be used in infected wounds and active against *Staphylococcus aureus, Streptococcus and Pseudomonas.*
- Polymyxin B sulphate-Gramicidin cream is similar to that above except it is also effective against *MRSA.*
- Silver sulfadiazine (2-7%) is frequently used in burn treatment and has a strong antimicrobial action against *Staphylococcus aureus, MRSA, Streptococcus, and Pseudomonas.*
- Silver (ionized), prepared in absorbent sheets and activated with sterile water, is effective against the same organisms as silver sulfadiazine. The moist environment increases reepithelialization.

Support surfaces

<u>Functions</u>
Support surfaces must provide a number of different functions:
- Temperature control is important because increases can lead to skin breakdown. Skin temperature relates to specific heat of the material in the support surface. Specific heat (the ability to conduct heat) varies considerably from one type of material to another. Air has a low specific

heat; and water, a high specific heat. Material with high specific heat may conduct heat away from the body, decreasing skin temperature.

- Moisture control prevents moisture damage to skin, but there are wide ranges of materials in use in support surfaces. Some materials, such as rubber or plastic, may increase perspiration and moisture, while some porous materials, such as some foams, may reduce perspiration.
- Friction/shear control is more difficult to achieve although some surface coverings, such as those with Gortex®, are purposely slick to decrease friction. However, proper positioning, lifting, and repositioning still must be done.

Pressure redistribution occurs through immersion (spreading the pressure out) and envelopment (conforming to shape without increasing pressure). The aim is to reduce pressure on the skin to less than the capillary closing pressure (<32mm Hg.), but lower pressures may be necessary for elderly patients. Interface pressure measurement is measurement of the pressure exerted between the body and the support surface. This measurement is currently used to evaluate the pressure redistribution efficiency of devices although it has not been demonstrates through research that this measurement can predict clinical performance. Thin, flexible sensors are placed under the support surface and patient and computerized readings indicate if the support surface is adequate. A number of new measurement devices are now marketed that show colored-coded computerized pictures demonstrating different levels of pressure.

General use guidelines to prevent pressure ulcers
A support surfaces redistributes pressure to prevent pressure ulcers and reduce shear and friction. There are various types of support surfaces for beds, examining tables, operating tables, and chairs. General use guidelines include:

- Pressure redistribution support surfaces should be used in beds, operating and examining tables for at-risk individuals.
- Patients with multiple ulcers, stage II or stage IV ulcers require support surfaces.
- Chairs should have gel or air support surfaces to redistribute pressure for chair bound patients, critically ill patients, or those who cannot move independently.
- Support surface material should provide at least an inch of support under areas to be protected when in use to prevent "bottoming out." (Check by placing hand palm-up under overlay below the pressure point.)
- Static support surfaces are appropriate for patients who can change position without increasing pressure to an ulcer.
- Dynamic support surfaces are needed for those who need assistance to move or when static pressure devices provide less than an inch of support.

Categories

There are 5 elements that are used to categorize support surfaces:

- Pressure redistribution may be preventive ($\leq$ 32mg Hg, but not consistently) or therapeutic (<32 mg Hg, consistently). Preventive devices are used for those at risk or with stage I or II ulcers. Therapeutic devices are used for those with stage III and IV pressure ulcers.
- Device forms are varied and may supplement or replace existing equipment. Devices include chair cushions, mattress overlays, pressure-reducing mattresses, and specialty bed systems used in place of traditional hospital beds.
- Power sources are powered, requiring attachment to an electrical motor for utilization, (dynamic) or non-powered (static).
- Medium may be different types of foam, water, gels, or air.
- Medicare reimbursement group:
  - Group 1: Used as a preventive measure and includes overlays and mattresses.
  - Group 2: Used as a therapeutic measure and includes non-powered or powered overlays and mattresses.
  - Group 3: Used as a therapeutic measure and includes air-fluidized beds.

Redistribution medium

Water

Water in overlays or mattresses is a common redistribution medium. The water may flow between cells or may be in one large space. Weight floating on water is evenly distributed, so waterbeds provide good weight distribution and they have good immersion qualities, so the patient's body sinks into the surface, which then molds to the body shape. While these devices are popular in the home, there are a number of disadvantages to their use in healthcare facilities:

- They require electricity and a heater to keep the correct temperature.
- Water is very heavy, so they are difficult to move and maneuver.
- Draining and filling is messy and time-consuming.
- They may leak if punctured or around connections.
- Water is pulled by gravity, so if the head of the bed is elevated, the water flows downward, leaving uneven distribution.
- Moving or repositioning patients on a water support surface can be difficult because of the constant movement of the water.

Foam

Foam varies considerably according to density and indentation load definition (ILD). Foam can be closed-cell (resistant) or open cell (visco-elastic). The number of chemicals used in manufacture of polyurethane foam determines the weight and visco-elasticity. Higher densities have higher visco-elastic (molding) properties. Open-cell foam is temperature-sensitive, helping it to mold to the body as it reaches the patient's body temperature. The density number of foam indicates the weight per cubic foot. Firmness is determined by the ILD, which is the number of pounds of pressure needed to indent a 4-inch foam 25% of its thickness using an indentation of 50 square inches. (Body weight and pounds of pressure should not be confused.) Foam is relatively inexpensive and was one of the first support surfaces used. Overlays should be 3-4 inches thick with densities of 1.3-1.6, and ILD of about 30. Foam has some disadvantages:

- Increases skin temperature.
- Has a short life-span
- Loses fire-retardance if it gets wet.

Air

Non-powered (static) air redistribution devices are manufactured in various forms: cushions, pads, overlays, and mattresses. The airfilled overlays may have single bladder or multi-cells/cylinders, with multi-cell forms providing the most pressure redistribution. Most forms are reusable and are filled with pumps to levels prescribed by the manufacturer according to the size and weight of the individual. The air moves with the individual, and the degree of immersion determines the effectives of the device. Powered (dynamic) alternating pressure overlays have cells or cylinders that are alternately inflated and deflated at prescribed intervals by way of a pump that is attached to the overlay. Air overlays must be checked frequently to ensure that there is adequate air filling. Disadvantages include susceptibility to shear when the bed is elevated and bottoming out. Air overlays are recommended only for those <250 pounds. The degree of temperature and moisture control depends on the covering.

Air-fluidized (high air loss) beds are special bed systems that have a high flow of air through silicon beads, originally designed for treatment of burn patients. As the air flows through the beads, it "fluidizes" them so that they move, and provide support and redistribution of pressure in much the way water does. The beads are contained in a bathtub-like frame. The lower part of the body becomes immersed in the beads so that the person appears to be floating as the beads move about because of the air. The air-fluidized bed is most commonly used for patients with multiple pressure ulcers, making positioning to avoid pressure on sores very difficult, or who have had surgery for myocutaneous flaps. These expensive beds provide a warm alkaline environment and a bactericidal effect, there is some indication that capillary perfusion may become occluded, resulting in pressure ulcers, although existing ulcers heal faster.

Low air loss beds, overlays, and cushions have porous surfaces that allow air that is pumped in the support surface to leak, so there is a continuous flow of air through the air pillows in the device. The air pressure in the pillows in the devices can be adjusted according to the individual needs. The low air loss bed systems provide better immersion than air overlays and the patient cannot bottom out if the device is properly maintained. The covers for the devices are usually made of nylon or

- 64 -

polytetrafluoroethylene fabric, which minimize friction. Only linen coverings or special pads that are air-permeable should be used with low air loss devices so that the air can flow beneath the skin. Disadvantages are that the equipment is expensive and contraindicated for those with an unstable spine. The airflow in beds must be maintained properly or there is a danger of "entrapment" in the bed. Hypothermia sometimes occurs.

<u>Gels</u>
Gels, which consist of silicone elastomer, silicone, or polyvinyl chloride, are fluid emulsions used in the manufacture of numerous devices, such as chair cushions and other types of flotation pads, such as overlays for beds, operating tables, beds, and exam tables. There are also gel mattress replacements. Gel flotation pads usually have covers that can be disinfected so they can be used by multiple patients, a factor in their versatility. They are relatively inexpensive and require no electricity. Gels provide protection against shear and have good immersion properties, molding well to the body shape and providing good pressure redistribution. There are, however, some disadvantages:
- They are heavy.
- The gel filling may break up over time, leading to uneven distribution.
- They are difficult to repair.
- They may increase body temperature.
- They are not suitable for moisture control.

Measures to promote mobility

Mobility is a problem for many patients with pressure ulcers because their restricted mobility is often the cause of the ulcers in the first place. However, promoting mobility to the extent possible improves circulation, aids healing, and decreases risk of developing further pressure ulcers:
- Bed bound patients must be repositioned on a scheduled basis and should receive passive ROM exercises and active bed exercises if tolerated daily. The patient's head should be elevated only to 30° for short periods of time.
- Patients with limited mobility should be evaluated by physical and occupational therapists in order to develop an individualized plan for activities. Patients may need assistive devices, such as walkers, canes, or wheelchairs. Because the wound must be protected without compromise to circulation, the amount and type of mobility or exercises related to the area and stage of the ulcer as well as underlying pathology or co-morbid conditions.

Measures to reduce pressure

Measures to reduce pressure include turning and repositioning.
- Goals for repositioning and a turning schedule of at least every 2 hours should be established for each individual, with documentation required.
- Devices, such as pillows or foam, should be used to correctly position patients so that bony prominences are protected and not in direct contact with each other.
- Re-position patients carefully to avoid friction or shear.
- Assistive devices should be used if necessary to move patients.
- Use chairs of correct size and height and pressure relieving devices for the seats.
- Limit chair time for those who are acutely ill to no more than 2 hours.
- Patients should be taught or reminded to redistribute weight every 15 minutes. A timer may be used to remind patients.
- Use the 30° lateral position rather than 90° side lying position.
- Use protective and support devices as needed.
- Avoid positioning on ulcers.

Measures for control of shear and friction

Because shear and friction are primary factors in development of pressure ulcers, measures to reduce them are essential:
- The head of the bed should never be elevated more than 30°; however, if bed bound patients may not be able to feed themselves at this angle. If the bed is elevated higher, the patient should be carefully positioned, using a pull sheet or overhead trapeze to make sure the patient is at the right position. The bed should be lowered as soon as possible.
- Making sure that the skin is dry and using fine cornstarch-based powders may help prevent the skin from "sticking" to the sheets.
- Pull sheets or mechanical lifting devices should be used to lift, move, or transfer the patient.
- Medical treatments may reduce restlessness.
- Heel and elbow protectors provide protection.

Note: elevating the foot of the bed to prevent sliding and shear simply increases pressure to the sacrococcygeal area, solving one problem by creating another.

Off-loading for neuropathic/diabetic ulcers

Because neuropathic ulcers are the most common cause of amputation, healing ulcers is of primary importance, so off-loading measures to relieve pressure on the wounds are often instituted:
- Total contact casts (TCC) encase the lower extremity in a walking cast that equalizes pressure of the plantar surface. The casts may have windows over pressure ulcers to allow observation and treatment. TCC is more successful than other off-loading measures, possibly because people restrict activity more.
- Removable cast walkers allow patients to remove the casts, but studies show that people only use them 28% of the time, decreasing effectiveness.
- Half shoes may have a high walking heel with the front of the foot elevated off of the ground. They often have Velcro closures.
- Bed rest prevents dependency or pressure.
- Wheelchairs allow dependency of limb but prevent pressure.
- Crutches/ walkers allow people some mobility but reduce pressure to extremity.
- Foam dressings provide cushioning.

Charcot's arthropathy

Charcot's arthropathy is the direct result of neuropathy that weakens the muscles of the foot and reduces sensations. The neuropathy weakens the muscles supporting the bones, which in turn become weak and fracture easily. Because of the lack of sensation, the patient may be unaware of the fracture and continue to walk, causing further deformity. The foot becomes inflamed and swollen with increased temperature in foot, but usually there is no pain. In time, the joint dislocation causes the arch to collapse. Treatment includes:
- Compression bandages for 2-3 weeks to reduce edema and inflammation.
- Total contact or non-weight-bearing cast applied for up to 9 months.
- Gradual weight bearing after skin has resumed normal temperature.
- Electrostimulation of the bone may improve healing.
- Medications, such as Fosamax® and Aredia® may be used to decrease bone destruction.
- Gradual weight bearing is resumed as foot temperature improves.

Adequacy of footwear for those with LEND

Examining footwear to determine if the fit is correct and if they are appropriate:
- Examine shoes and slippers for bulges on the side that may indicate the shoes are too tight, wear patterns on the shoes or heels that may indicate uneven gait or weight distribution. Check inside the shoes to see if there is worn or torn lining that could irritate the skin. Make sure that there is

adequate cushioning. Sandals and open-toed shoes should be avoided because of the potential for foot injury.
- Foot imprints: Using the Harris Mat®, the patient steps down barefoot on the mat that creates a visual (inked) image of the foot, showing pressure areas with darker images. It shows areas of the foot at greatest risk.
- Forefoot test: An outline of both bare feet is traced on paper while the patient is standing if possible. Then the shoes are placed over this and another outline drawn. The entire foot outline should be inside the shoe outline.

Pulsed lavage

Pulsed lavage (pulsatile high pressure lavage) is irrigation of an infected or necrotic wound under pressure, using an electrically powered device. Normal saline is commonly used for lavage treatments with the amount varying according to the size and amount of exudate on the wound.   It is recommended that pressure be between 8-15 psi. The pressure can be varied as needed. While there is concern that higher pressure may inoculate tissue with bacteria, studies have not indicated this. Exposed blood vessels, graft sties, and muscle tissue should be avoided with the lavage treatments, and treatments should be discontinued if bleeding occurs with patients taking anticoagulants. Treatment is usually done 1 or 2 times daily. Both the hose and irrigating nozzle are intended for one-time use, so treatments can be expensive. Because of possible mist contamination, the treatment must be done in a separate enclosed space, and staff must wear personal protective equipment.

Hydrotherapy

Hydrotherapy, often in the form of whirlpool treatments to a limb or the whole body, is used to cleanse and debride wounds that are large with significant necrosis. Hydrotherapy is frequently used to treat burn injuries. Water is used at a temperature of 37°C. Antiseptics are sometimes added to the water, but these can interfere with healing. Hydrotherapy has been implicated in a number of outbreaks of wound infections caused by cross-contamination; so many facilities have discontinued the use of whirlpools. Additionally, they are contraindicated for venous ulcers because vasodilation can increase edema. Diabetic patients may be insensitive to temperature, so therapy must be used cautiously. Wounds related to arterial insufficiency may not benefit. Whirlpool treatments do not appear to reduce surface bacteria of wounds, but rinsing the tissue after the treatment does. Equipment must be thoroughly disinfected between patients to prevent spread of infection.

Autolytic debridement

Autolysis takes advantage of the body's enzymes and white blood cells to debride the wound by using proteolytic, fibrinolytic, and collagenolytic enzymes to soften and liquefy slough and eschar. Autolysis takes place in a warm, moist environment with adequate vasculature to provide white blood cells and neutrophil, so the neutrophil count must be adequate (>500mm³) or sepsis can occur. Autolysis is most successful in stage III or IV uninfected wounds and when exudate is light to moderate so that occlusive dressings can be maintained. Autolysis does not damage the periwound tissue, and it is an easy method of debridement, causing very little discomfort; however, it is slower than some methods, taking 72-96 hours before effects are demonstrated. Autolysis may be combined with other types of debridement, using autolysis first to soften and loosen eschar. Autolysis requires close monitoring of the wound, which may appear to enlarge as the eschar dissolves, showing the true dimensions of the wound.

Autolytic debridement requires a warm, moist, atmosphere, so occlusive or semi-occlusive dressings must be applied to the wound area. All moisture-retentive dressings promote autolysis to some degree, even when other methods of debridement are used, but as a sole means of debridement, it is recommended only for relatively small, uninfected wounds. The dressings most commonly used for autolytic debridement include:
- Hydrocolloids provide absorbency for wounds with small amounts of exudate, but may promote anaerobic infections if the dressing is occlusive.
- Alginate dressings provide added absorbency for wounds with large amounts of exudate, but require a secondary dressing to secure.
- Hydrogels are particularly helpful when wounds are dry because they add necessary moisture and promote rapid autolysis.
- Transparent films promotes autolysis for very small, shallow wounds or when used as a secondary dressing.

As the wound debrides, odor and drainage increases, so periwound tissue must be protected from exudate.

Enzymatic debridement

Enzymatic debridement is a method of chemical debridement that can be used on any type of wound that has a large amount of necrosis and eschar, especially chronic wounds and burns. Enzymes either directly digest the fibrin, bacteria, leukocytes, and other cell debris that comprises slough or dissolves the collagen that secures it to the wound. Enzymes need a moist environment, so if enzymes are used to debride dry eschar, the eschar must be crosshatched through the upper layers with a scalpel to allow the enzymes to penetrate the eschar. Enzymes are selective and do not damage viable tissue although some people have local irritation from the enzymes, particularly if the enzyme contains papain. Enzymatic debridement is relatively fast-acting but can still take days to weeks to complete debridement, especially with large wounds, so it is slower than some other techniques.

Enzymatic debridement uses chemical enzymes. Enzymes can be used with any type of dressing, but the enzymes need to be applied to necrotic tissue 1-2 times daily, so long-term dressings are not cost-effective. Moisture-retentive dressings speed debridement. Two types of enzyme preparations are used:

- Collagenase (Santyl®), derived from Clostridium bacteria, digests denatured collagen and is administered once daily by tongue blade into deep wounds or applied to gauze for shallow wounds. It is inactivated by low pH (optimum range is 6-8) hexachlorophene and heavy metal ions, including mercury, zinc, silver, as well as Burrow's solution.
- Papain/urea combinations (Accuzyme®, Panafil White®, Panafil®, Gladase®), derived from papaya, with or without chlorophyllin copper complex sodium, which reduces inflammation and odor. This enzyme digests nonviable protein composing the necrotic tissue. It is applied 1-2 times daily and is inactivated by hydrogen peroxide and salts of heaving metals, including lead, silver and mercury. It works at a pH of 3-12.

Biological debridement with maggots

Maggot debridement is inexpensive, faster than other non-surgical therapies, and effective, but is usually saved for cases not responding well to other therapy. Sterilized maggots (blowfly larvae) secrete proteolytic enzymes, including collagenase, which debrides the wound, as well as growth factors and cytokines, which increase healing. The teeth of the maggots penetrate the eschar, aiding the enzymes. While the FDA has approved Medical Maggots® only for debridement, numerous reports indicate that they also are effective against wound infections, such as MRSA. Antibiotics are often given concurrently with infected wounds because maggots can pickup pathogens in the wound and spread them in the tissue and to the bloodstream. Maggots are effective for many wounds, including pressure and stasis ulcers and burns. Maggots cannot be used with hydrogels. Periwound tissue must be protected from exudate. Large numbers of maggots should not be used in areas where blood vessels are exposed or damaged to prevent bleeding. Those on anticoagulants must be observed for bleeding.

Medical Maggots® are applied to the open wound; periwound tissue must be protected:

- A wound pattern is transferred onto a hydrocolloid pad, opening cut, and pad applied to the skin with the wound exposed. The pattern is used to cut an opening in a semi-permeable film for an outer dressing.
- Maggots are wiped from the container with a saline-dampened 2X2 gauze (about 5-10 maggots per cm^2 wound size). The gauze is loosely packed into the wound.
- A porous mesh (Creature Comfort®) is placed over the wound and secured to the hydrocolloid with tape or glue, creating a maggot cage.

- Transparent film is placed over the hydrocolloid, making sure that the cutout area is over the cage so that the maggots have air and drainage can escape. Saline-dampened gauze is placed loosely over cage.
- Dry gauze is used for the outer dressing and changed every 4-8 hours as needed.
- Maggots are wiped from the wound after 48 hours and wound irrigated with normal saline.

Mechanical debridement

Wet to dry
Wet-to-dry debridement is a common treatment in use for many years to debride wounds and absorb exudate, but it is non-selective in that it can pull healthy and granulating tissue from wounds as well. Treatment usually involves applying saline-moistened gauze to a wound and allowing it to dry for 4-6 hours and then pulling it off the wound. Using this approach to removing necrosis tissue can take days to weeks, depending upon the extent of the wound. It's important in wet-to-dry debridement that the dressings dry out completely, so the dressing should be moist but not saturated. One major drawback to wet-to-dry debridement is that it is quite painful, but wetting the gauze prior to removal to ease the pain decreases the effectiveness. This method requires frequent dressing changes and careful aseptic technique. Most experts in wound care no longer recommend wet-to-dry debridement or advise it only initially for heavily necrotic wounds.

Sharp
Sharp (instrumental) debridement involves the cutting away of necrotic tissue using forceps, scissors, and a scalpel. This is the most aggressive form of debridement that can be done by non-physician medical personnel, and regulations about doing this therapy vary from state to state. In some states, it is in the scope of practice for RNs while in other states it is within the scope of physical therapist's duties. Sharp debridement cleans the wound much faster than other non-surgical forms of debridement, promoting faster healing, and is selective as the person doing the debridement controls the type and amount of tissue that is removed. Procedure involves:
- Using aseptic technique and sterile equipment
- Cleansing the site of debridement with an antiseptic
- Holding the tissue taut with forceps to establish a plane of dissection.
- Dissecting carefully, avoiding vasculature.
- Irrigating the wound with normal saline upon completion.

Surgical debridement

Surgical debridement is instrumental dissection of necrotic tissue under general, spinal, or local anesthesia. It is most commonly used when very large amounts of tissue must be debrided, such as with extensive burns, or when there is a serious infection and immediate debridement is needed in order to effectively treat the wound infection. General anesthesia allows extensive debridement to be done without the patient suffering associated pain and trauma although postoperative pain is common. One advantage is that most debridement can be done in one procedure. Surgical debridement has been shown to stimulate healing in diabetic ulcers. However, there are risks associated with anesthesia and post-operative wound infections can occur. It is also much more costly than other methods. An alternative surgical method is laser debridement, which can cut away necrotic tissue. Pulsed laser beams are less damaging to adjacent tissue than continuous lasers.

Chemical cauterization

Chemical cauterization with silver nitrate is sometimes used to treat hypergranulation. Cauterization uses heat to burn or sear abnormal cells in order to destroy them. Silver nitrate sticks are wet with water to activate and are then gently rolled over the tissue to be treated for a short time. Chemical cauterization is used infrequently, for such things as treatment of nosebleeds and warts. The most common uses for chemical cauterization in wounds or skin lesions are to control hypergranulation tissue that grows in wounds, especially about stomas or to treat warts. Hypergranulation is excessive soft flaccid granulating tissue that is raised above the level of the periwound tissue, preventing proper epithelization, and may reflect excess moisture in the wound. Hypergranulation tissue is often friable and bleeds easily. It may produce both exudates that interfere with healing and odor. Treatment may be repeated 2 times daily for 1-4 days until excess tissue sloughs.

Improving perfusion

There are a number of measures than can improve perfusion of wounds in order to promote wound healing:
- Smoking cessation to reduce vascular constriction.
- Monitoring glucose and controlling blood glucose levels with diet and medication.
- Controlling high blood pressure with diet and medications.
- Reducing lipid levels through diet and medications.
- Aspirin therapy to reduce danger of clot formation.
- Surgical revascularization to replace damaged vessels.
- Hyperbaric oxygen therapy increases available oxygen to tissues by 10-20 times. Blood that is saturated increases perfusion of the tissues. It is indicated for peripheral arterial insufficiency, compromised skin from grafts, and diabetic ulcers.
- Topical hyperbaric oxygen therapy (THOT®) has shown promise in increasing circulation and healing wounds. The topical oxygen increases perfusion to the wound bed itself rather than systemically.

- Circulator Boot® therapy, an end-diastolic compression equipment system is used to treat ulcers of the lower extremity. Compressions coordinate with the end of diastole to increase perfusion. It is FDA approved for the treatment of deficient arterial blood flow.

Hyperbaric oxygen treatments

Hyperbaric oxygen therapy (HBOT) is treatment in a high pressure chamber while breathing 100% oxygen, which increases available oxygen to tissues by 10-20 times. Blood that is saturated increases perfusion of the tissues. HBOT has shown considerable promise in reducing the need for amputation resulting from ulcerations of the lower extremities, but it is critical that treatment be instituted early enough while the potential for salvage remains. HBOT is used for a number of conditions, but is especially important for hypoxic wounds, such as those associated with peripheral arterial insufficiency, compromised skin from grafts, and diabetic ulcers. Treatment protocols vary according to the type of wound, but are limited to 90 minutes to avoid oxygen toxicity. HBOT has the following effects:
- Hyperoxygenation of blood and tissue.
- Vasoconstriction, reducing capillary leakage.
- Angiogenesis because of increased fibroblasts and collagen.
- Increased antibiotic effectiveness for those needing active transport. Across cell walls (fluoroquinolone, amphotericin B, aminoglycosides).

Negative pressure wound therapy

Negative pressure wound therapy (NPWT) uses subatmospheric (negative) pressure with a suction unit and a semi-occlusion vapor-permeable dressing. The suction reduces periwound and interstitial edema, decompressing vessels and improving circulation. It also stimulates production of new cells and decreases colonization of bacteria. NPWT also increases the rate of granulation and re-epithelialization so that wounds heal more quickly. The wound must be debrided of necrotic tissue prior to treatment.

NPWT is used for a variety of difficult to heal wounds, especially those that show less than 30% healing in 4 weeks of post-debridement treatment or those with excessive exudate:
- Chronic stage II and IV pressure ulcers.
- Skin flaps.
- Diabetic ulcers.
- Acute wounds.
- Burns, both partial and full-thickness.
- Unresponsive arterial and venous ulcers.
- Surgical wounds and those with dehiscence.

It is contraindicated in some conditions:
- Wound malignancy
- Untreated osteomyelitis
- Exposed blood vessels or organs
- Nonenteric, unexplored fistulas.

Application of negative pressure wound therapy is done after the wound is determined to be appropriate for this treatment and debridement is completed, leaving the wound tissue exposed. There are a number of different electrical suction NPWT systems, such as the VAC® (vacuum-assisted closure) system and the Versatile I® (VI). Application steps include:
- Apply nonadherent porous foam cut to fit and completely cover the wound
  - Polyurethane (hydrophobic, repelling moisture) is used for all wounds EXCEPT those that are painful, have tunneling or sinus tracts, deep trauma wounds, and wounds needing controlled growth of granulation.
  - Polyvinyl (hydrophilic), is used for all wound EXCEPT deep wounds with moderate granulation, deep pressure ulcers and flaps.
- Secure foam occlusive transparent film.
- Cut opening to accommodate the drainage tube in the dressing and attach drainage tube.
- Attach tube to suction canister, creating closed system.
- Set pressure to 75-125, as indicated.
- Change dressings 2-3 times weekly.

Growth factor treatments

Growth factors are proteins that are necessary for growth and migration of cells, and are thus critical elements in healing of wounds. Growth factors may be isolated from tumor cells, platelets, macrophages, ovarian follicles, and the placenta, but recombinant DNA techniques have allowed production of synthetic growth factor from bacterial cultures or human cells with the growth factor genes. Growth factors are applied topically to the wound. There are a number of different types of growth factors in use or study, including:
- Connective Tissue Growth Factor (CTGF) is being studied for use to combat fibrosis.
- Epidermal Growth Factor (EGF) is used for burns and venous ulcers.
- Fibroblast Growth Factor (FGF) is used for burns and pressure ulcers.
- Insulin-Like Growth Factor (IGF) is being studied as a means to reduce HbAIC in diabetes.
- Platelet-Derived Growth Factor (PDGF) is used for pressure and diabetic ulcers.
- Transforming Growth Factor-Beta (TGF-β) is used with chronic skin ulcers.

Static compression therapy

Static compression therapy is applying external graduated pressure to lower extremity, from the ankle to the knee to support the calf muscle and increase venous flow. Compression therapy is not curative, but is used as a preventive and therapeutic treatment to eliminate edema. It is contraindicated in those with heart failure or peripheral arterial disease as it may further impair compromised arterial circulation. Compression should not be used if the ankle brachial index (ABI) is <0.5. There are many different types of static compression products, and they should be chosen according to individual needs. They are graded according to the level of compression:

- High level provides therapeutic compression at 30-40 mmHg at the ankle. Some may provide pressure at 40-50 mmHg. ABI should be >0.8.
- Low level provides modified pressure up to 23mmHg at the ankle. ABI must be >0.5 to <0.8. While this level is less than therapeutic, some authorities believe that even low levels of pressure provide some therapeutic benefit.

<u>Elastic</u>
There are many products and different types of elastic static compression therapy:

- Layered wraps (Profore®, ProGuide®, and Dynapress®) combine both elastic and non-elastic layers in 2-4 layers with the inner layers providing protection to bony prominences and absorbing drainage. Different products require different wrapping methods, spiral or figure-8. The skin is usually lubricated to prevent drying. These are used for both ambulatory and non-ambulatory patients. The dressing must be applied by a professional and are changed 1-2 times weekly. Layered wraps are frequently used for early treatments. Some wraps have visual pressure indicators.
- Single-layer wraps (SurePress®) are long reusable elastic wraps that are used for early treatment or maintenance and can be used by both ambulatory and non-ambulatory patients. Competent caregivers can be taught to apply these dressings, especially those with visual pressure indicators. Because they are reusable, they are more cost effective than single-use dressings.
- Therapeutic compression stockings (Jobst®, Juzo®, Sig-Varis®, Medi-Strumpf®, Therapress Duo®) are used to prevent ulceration in those with varicose veins and stable venous insufficiency after edema is controlled or with existing ulcers when edema recedes. They are contraindicated with lipodermatosclerosis because of the difficulty fitting the stocking. They may be used for both ambulatory and non-ambulatory patients who are able to apply the stockings. The stockings come in many sizes and colors and may extend from the foot to the knee or the groin. The stockings must be fitted properly and have the correct level of compression:
    - Class I: 20-30 mm Hg (varicose veins)
    - Class 2: 30-40 mm Hg (venous ulcers and prevention)
    - Class 3: 40-50 mm Hg (refractory venous ulcers & lymphedema)
    - Class 4: 50-60 mm Hg (lymphedema)

Non-elastic orthotics

The CircAid Thera-Boot® is a stocking with multiple Velcro straps so that it can be adjusted to fit. The straps make adjusting easy for patients or caregivers. The ankle-foot wrap is attached to cover the foot and ankle but is thin enough to fit into a standard shoe. The orthotic provides continuous compression as well as supporting the calf muscle pump function. The orthotic comes in three sizes (small, medium, and large) according to ankle and calf measurement. It is washable and reusable and can adjust to changes in limb size, so it is more cost-effective than some other devices. Also, it can be adjusted as needed during activities. The CircAid Thera-Boot® was designed specifically for treatment of venous ulcers, but should not be used until edema has subsided. It can be used initially for treatment as well as for maintenance.

Non-elastic

There are many products and different types of non-elastic static compression therapy:

- Unna's boot (ViscoPaste®) is a gauze wrap impregnated with zinc oxide, glycerin, or gelatin to provide a supporting compression "boot" to provide support to the calf muscle pump during ambulation, so they are not suitable for non-ambulatory patients. They can be used for those with peripheral arterial disease. The bandage must be applied carefully without tension. It may be left open to dry or covered with an elastic or self-adherent wrap. The dressings are changed according to the individual needs, determined by a decrease in edema, the amount of exudate, and hygiene with dressing changes ranging from 2 times weekly to every other week.
- Short-stretch wrap (Comprilan®) is reusable and indicated for ambulatory patients and those with borderline ABIs (>0.5-<0.8). It is used for both initial and maintenance therapy. Caregivers can be taught to apply, but dressings slip out of place easily.

IPC therapy

Intermittent pneumatic compression (IPC) therapy is indicated if static compression therapy is ineffective or the patient is immobile. (Medicare reimbursement requires a 6- month trial of static compression therapy.) IPC devices are used on the lower leg or plantare area of the foot. IPC devices have a garment and a pneumatic pump that inflates the garment. The device for the leg typically has a double-lined stocking that fits over the leg. One lining contains an air bladder with segments so that the intermittent inflations occur segmentally up the leg, increasing venous return. The foot pump takes advantage of the physiologic pumping function in the sole of the foot to stimulate blood flow. The Circulator Boot® is an end-diastolic IPC that is timed to the end of diastole to improve arterial flow while improving venous return. Treatments are usually 1-2 times daily for 1-2 hours and decrease edema and promote healing of ulcers. IPC therapy is contraindicated for those with uncompensated heart failure, for those with active thrombus.

Sickle cell diseases and thalassemia

Sickle cell diseases comprise a group of inherited hemolytic blood disorders that result in destruction of hemoglobin and misshapen "sickle-shaped" cells that tend to cluster together, occluding vessels and causing severe pain. Ulcerations may result, usually on the malleolus of a lower extremity. There may be single or multiple lesions, varying in size, associated with edema and slow healing. Treatment includes:
- Reducing edema with elevation, compression, and bed rest.
- Controlling the disease through medications or transfusions.
- Moisture-retentive dressings to promote healing.
- Debridement as indicated.
- Monitoring for infection.

Thalassemia is an inherited disease that results in abnormal hemoglobin and microcytic anemia. It most often occurs in those of Mediterranean descent. Because the hemoglobin carries less iron, patients are more susceptible to trauma and tissue damage. Treatment includes:
- Moisture-retentive dressings and prevention of wound hypothermia.
- Controlling the disease with blood transfusions and iron-chelation therapy.
- Protecting wound from further trauma.

Topical therapy for surgical wounds

Topical therapy for surgical wounds is generally conservative, observing for signs of healing and infection. The standard use of antimicrobials and antiseptics is generally not indicated because of the danger of resistance and the cytotoxic properties of some that delay healing. Therapy includes:
- Initial dressing to provide protection and absorb any exudate as well as to provide thermal insulation to promote healing. Dressings should be lightly applied in order to prevent compression that may impede perfusion to the wound. These may be left in place for 48-72 hours to allow the wound to begin to seal.
- If there are signs of local infection, a topical antimicrobial (such as Neosporin®) or antiseptic (such as povidone iodine) may be applied to the surgical incision site.
- Depending upon the site of the incision, after the initial healing has taken place, the wound may be left uncovered or a soft dressing may be kept in place to prevent local irritation.

Management of tissue damage related to contact dermatitis

Contact dermatitis is a localized response to contact with an allergen, resulting in a rash that may blister and itch. Common allergens include poison oak, poison ivy, latex, benzocaine, nickel, and preservatives, but there is a wide range of items preparations and products to which people may react. Treatment includes:
- Identifying the causative agent through evaluating the area of the body affected, careful history, or skin patch testing to determine allergic responses.
- Corticosteroids to control inflammation and itching.
- Soothing oatmeal baths.
- Caladryl® lotion to relieve itching.
- Antihistamines to reduce allergic response.
- Lesions should be gently cleansed and observed for signs of secondary infection.
- Antibiotics are used only for secondary infections as indicated.
- Rash is usually left open to dry.
- Avoidance of allergen will prevent recurrence.

Traumatic wounds

Spider bites
Spider bites are frequently a misdiagnosis of a *Staphylococcus aureus* or MRSA infection, so unless the spider was observed, the wound should be cultured and antibiotics started. If the wound responds to the antibiotic, then it probably wasn't a spider bite. There are 2 main types of venomous spider bites:
- Producing neurological symptoms (Black widow).
- Producing local necrosis (brown recluse, yellow sac and hobos spiders).

Treatment includes:
- Cleanse wound and apply cool compress and elevate body part if possible.
- Black widow bites:
    o Narcotic analgesics.
    o Nitroprusside to relieve hypertension.
    o Calcium gluconate 10% solution IV for abdominal cramps.
    o Latrodectus antivenin for those with severe reaction.
- Necrotic/ulcerated bites (brown recluse, etc.).
    o There is no consensus on the best treatment as ulceration caused by the venom may be extensive and surgical repair with grafts may be needed.
    o Treatment as for other necrotic ulcers, with moisture retentive dressings as indicated.
    o Hyperbaric oxygen therapy (HBOT) has been used in some cases.

Animal bites

There is no one topical therapy for traumatic wounds because they vary so widely in the type and degree of injury. A scrape on the knee is treated very differently from a car accident that involves massive tissue injury or tissue loss. Animal bites, including human, are frequent causes of traumatic injury. Treatment includes:

- Cleanse wound by flushing with 10-35cc syringe with 18-gauge angiocath to remove debris and bacteria using normal saline or dilute Betadine® solution.
- Hand, puncture, and infected wounds or those more than 12 hours old may be closed by secondary intention.
- Moisture-retentive dressings as indicated by the size and extent of injury of wound left open. Dry dressings may be applied to injuries with closure by primary intention.
- Topical antibiotics may be indicated although systemic antibiotics are commonly prescribed for animal bites.
- Tetanus toxoid or immune globulin is routinely administered.

Snake bites

About 45,000 snake bites occur in the United States each year, with about 8000 poisonous. In the United States, about 25 species of snakes are venomous. There are 2 types of snakes that can cause serious injury, classified according to the type of fangs and venom. Coral snakes have short fixed permanent fangs in the upper jaw and venom that is primarily neurotoxic, but may also have hemotoxic and cardiotoxic properties:

- Wounds show no fang marks but there may be scratches or semi-circular markings from teeth.
- There may be little local reaction, but neurological symptoms may range from mild to acute respiratory and cardiovascular failure.
- Treatment includes:
- Cleansing wound thoroughly of dirt and debris and leave open or cover with dry dressing.
- Antibiotics not usually needed.
- Administering antivenin immediately even without symptoms, which may be delayed.
- Tetanus toxoid or immune globulin.

A second type that can cause serious injury are the pit vipers. Rattlesnakes, copperheads, and cottonmouths have erectile fangs that fold until they are aroused, and venom is primarily hemotoxic and cytotoxic but may have neurotoxic properties. Wounds usually show 1-2 fang marks. Edema may begin immediately or may be delayed up to 6 hours. Pain may be severe. There may be a wide range of symptoms, including hypotension and coagulopathy with defibrination that can lead to excessive blood loss, depending upon the type and amount of venom. There may be local infection and necrosis.

Treatment includes:
- Cleansing wound thoroughly and dressings as indicated.
- Tetanus toxoid or immune globulin.
- Analgesics, such as morphine sulphate
- Avoiding NSAIDs and aspirin because of anticoagulation properties.
- Marking edema every 15 minutes.
- Antivenin therapy if indicated (observation for serum sickness if horse serum used).
- Prophylactic antibiotics for severe tissue necrosis.
- Platelets, plasma, or packed RBCs for coagulopathy.

Alligator bites
Alligators are found in 10 coastal states in the southeastern United States with the largest population in Florida, where most injuries are reported. Animals between 4-8 feet often bite once and release, but larger animals may bite repeatedly, engaging in typical biting and feeding activities, and resulting in severe injury, amputations, or death. Most wounds involve the limbs, with the hands and arms the most frequently bitten. Treatment includes:
- Treatment for shock and blood loss.
- Applying pressure to wound.
- Retrieving amputated limbs if possible.
- Flushing wound with copious amounts of normal saline to reduce contamination.
- Wound cultures.
- Prophylactic broad-spectrum antibiotics for Gram negative organisms, such as *Aeromonas hydrophila* and *Clostridium.*
- Observation for signs of infection, such as erythema, cellulitis, exudate, necrosis).
- Tetanus toxoid or immune globulin.
- Repair of fractures.
- Surgical repair and debridement as indicated with wounds usually healing by secondary intention or delayed primary closure.

Autoimmune wounds

PV
Pemphigus vulgaris (PV) an autoimmune disorder causing blistering of both the skin and the mucous membranes (presenting symptom in 50-70% of patients), creates burn-like wounds, which may heal slowly or not at all, often starting in the mouth and genital areas. Untreated the disorder can lead to death. Blisters on skin rupture, causing ulcerations, and those in folds may develop hypergranulation and crusting. Treatment includes:
- Corticosteroids (Prednisone®) and immunosuppressive drugs (Imuron®).
- Nutritional assessment. Vit D and calcium supplement may be needed.
- Careful observation for secondary infections.

- Protective clothing and minimize trauma to skin.
- Rituxan®, a drug used for lymphoma and leukemia, has helped patients go into remission when used with other drugs.
- Talcum powder applied to sheets if lesions on back.
- Good oral care with soft toothbrush.
- Plasmapheresis with plasma removed to reduce antibodies and donated plasma infused.
- Potassium permanganate lotion bath (1:10000) and chlorhexidine tulle gauze dressing of the denuded areas.

Atypical ulcerations

Pyoderma granulosum
Pyoderma granulosum *is* a painful ulcerative condition of the skin that is often associated with underlying systemic diseases (such as inflammatory bowel disease) and dysregulation of immunity involving neutrophils. There are two types:
- Classical: deep ulcerations with border overhanging wound bed, most common on the legs, but may be about stomas.
- Atypical: vesicopustular draining lesions, usually on the top of the hands, the forearms, or face.

Treatment includes:
- Topical and systemic corticosteroids and systemic immunosuppressive drugs.
- Local wound care and dressings as indicated for the type and degree of wound, includes moisture-retentive non-adherent dressings.
- Autolysis is only debridement because of danger of extending the disease.
- Topical antibiotics may be necessary to control infection.
- Treating the underlying systemic cause, such as colectomy for ulcerative colitis, may reduce symptoms.
- Surgical treatment of lesions is usually avoided.

Epidermolysis bullosa
Epidermolysis bullosa (EB) comprises a group of inherited and non-inherited bullous (blistering) disorders of different levels of the epithelial tissue, with even mild mechanical trauma resulting in blistering. Symptoms vary widely and may range from slight seasonal blistering to life-threatening erosions of skin. It may affect internal epithelial tissue in mucous membranes and organs as well as the external dermal layers. There are different categories of EB:
- Simplex (EBS): intraepidermal lesions
- Junctional (JEB): Blistering at lamina lucida (between epidermis and basement membrane)

- Recessive dystrophic (RDEB): Separation at basement membrane. Excessive scarring and blistering from slight mechanical trauma, leading to hemorrhage and ulceration. Predisposes to squamous cell carcinoma.
- Dominant dystrophic (DDEB): Blisters below basement membrane with scarring. Less severe than RDEB.

Treatment includes:
- Nutritional assessment and supplements as needed.
- Topical antibiotics or silver-impregnated dressings for infection.
- Protection to avoid trauma.
- *Fenestrated non-adherent dressings, secured with stockinet, roll gauze, or tubular gauze.

Vasculitis

Vasculitis comprises a large number of disorders that result in inflammation of veins, arteries, and capillaries, causing changes in vessel walls. Symptoms vary widely, but frequently include fever, general malaise, myalgia, loss of appetite, and skin lesions. Skin lesions may range from macular rashes to large necrotic ulcerations. Lesions are commonly on the lower extremities and may be confused with venous lesions. Disorders that may cause vasculitis with hemorrhagic rash or ulcerations include Behcet's syndrome, Henoch-Schonlein purpura, rheumatoid vasculitis, systemic lupus erythematosus, polyarteritis nodosa, and Wegener's granulomatosis. Treatment includes:
- Medical control of underlying disease process.
- Systemic corticosteroids, antihistamines, and immunosuppressants.
- Debridement of necrosis.
- Observation for infection and treatment with topical or systemic antibiotics as indicated.
- Moisture retentive dressings with absorptive material if needed for exudate.
- Skin sealants or barriers to protect periwound tissue from exudate.
- Monitor nutrition and provide supplements as needed.

Toxic epidermal necrolysis

Toxic epidermal necrolysis is a rare life-threatening condition of the epidermis caused by drug reactions to 3 types of drugs: antibiotics (sulfonamides, allopurinol, and ampicillin), anticonvulsants (phenytoin, carbamazepine, and phenobarbital), and analgesics (acetaminophen and NSAIDS). An initial maculopapular rash gives way to erythema and painful skin that sloughs with the slightest pressure, leaving >10% of the body denuded of epidermis. The skin, mucous membranes, eyes, and respiratory tract may be involved with mortality rates of 30-40%.

Treatment includes:
- Surgical debridement of sloughing skin with saline-moistened cloth.
- Porcine xenografts stapled into place
- Patient placed in air-fluidized bed in burn unit.

- Fluid and electrolytes monitored and replaced.
- NG feedings
- Systemic antibiotics and cessation of any corticosteroids.
- Pain control with opioids.
- Pulmonary and ophthalmic care.
- Grafts trimmed as they desiccate and wounds heal.

Calciphylaxis

Calciphylaxis is a rare fatal disease related to end-stage renal disease and uremia, resulting in vascular calcification of cutaneous blood vessels and necrotic lesions with typical violet discoloration. Mortality rates range from 60-80%, usually caused by sepsis. Patients present with painful discolored lesions that progress to nodules and ulcerations that become infected and gangrenous. Lesions are most common in areas with accumulation of fatty tissue. Blood flow distal to the ulcerations is usually intact. The etiology is unclear, but it is associated with hypercalcemia, hyperphosphatemia, and hyperparathyroidism. Treatment is often palliative as there is no successful standardized approach although the disorder frequently results in amputation of the affected limb:
- Control of calcium and phosphorus levels.
- Intravenous sodium thiosulfate to reduce calcium deposits.
- Surgical or medical treatment of hyperparathyroidism.
- Antibiotics as indicated for wound infections
- Aggressive debridement with absorbent moisture-retentive dressings.
- Analgesia as indicated.

GVHD

Graft-versus-host disease (GVHD) is caused by a severe host reaction to bone marrow transplantation. Acute GVHD occurs within 100 days after surgery; and chronic, after 100 days. The skin, liver (causing jaundice and pruritis), and large and small intestines (causing bleeding and diarrhea) may all be involved. A maculopapular (red to violet) rash usually begins on the hands, plantar area of foot, face, and upper trunk, which spreads and may results in desquamation and formation of bullae. The disease is staged 1-4 depending on severity. Treatment includes:
- Colony-stimulating factor (CSF) for 6 months and other appropriate immunosuppressive therapy.
- Topical corticosteroids may be used.
- Careful observation and cleansing of skin for signs of infection.
- Severe denudement requires debridement and transfer to the burn unit for treatment appropriate to condition to prevent further deterioration.
- Adhesive occlusive dressings should be avoided.

Fungating neoplastic wounds

Fungating neoplastic wounds occur in up to 10% of those with metastasis, especially involving oral or breast caner. Fungating wounds are ulcerating with necrosis and slough and may have a foul odor and small to copious amount of drainage. Infection is common and the periwound tissue may become inflamed, macerated or tender. The prognosis is very poor and treatment may be primarily palliative, depending upon the condition of the patient:

- Control bleeding: the ulcers bleed as the vasculature erodes; so hemostatic dressings (Gel foam, alginates) and cauterization with silver nitrate may be necessary. Use non-adherent dressings or long-term dressings to reduce trauma.
- Manage exudate: Foam, alginate or hydrofiber dressings or wound pouch as indicated.
- Control odor: Use of charcoal dressing or Chloromycetin solution.
- Protect periwound tissue: Skin sealants, barrier ointments, and hydrocolloid waters to anchor tape.
- Cleanse wound: Use ionic cleansers or antiseptics.
- Control pain: Analgesia as indicated.

Tissue damage related to irradiation

<u>Staging</u>
Because the cells in the skin are constantly going through mitotic division, they are vulnerable to the effects of irradiation. Most reactions subside 1-3 months after therapy ends. Damage is staged according to the type and degree of reaction, and staging determines treatment:

- Stage I: Slight edema and inflammation with erythema that may result in burning, itching and discomfort, caused by dilation and increased permeability of capillaries
- Stage II: Dry, itching, scaly skin with partial sloughing of epidermis, caused by inability of basal epidermal cells to adequately replace surface cells and decreased functioning of skin glands.
- Stage III: Moist blistering skin with loss of epidermal tissue, serous drainage, and increased pain with exposure of nerves, caused by continued deterioration of skin.
- Stage IV: Loss of body hair and sweat gland suppression resulting in permanent hair loss, atrophy, pigment changes, and ulcerations, caused by accumulation of radiation in the tissues.

<u>Treatment</u>
Management of tissue damage related to irradiation focuses on treating damage and preventing deterioration in order to relieve discomfort and promote healing. Patients must be educated about the need for skin care during therapy:

- Protect skin by maintaining cleanliness, avoiding irritants, using electric razors, protecting from sunlight and extremes of heat and cold, apply appropriate emollients, using mild soaps, and wearing loose protective clothing.
- Relieve discomfort by using cornstarch or powders (NOT talcum) in dry areas, applying topical corticosteroids sparingly to reduce itching.
- Treat open areas by using saline compresses, Sitz baths, and semi-occlusive dressings as indicated to protect nerve endings. Prevent damage to wounds by using non-adherent dressings and securing them with mesh or stockinet instead of tape. Culture wounds and treat bacterial or fungus infections as indicated. Use dressings appropriate for the amount and type of exudate to prevent further skin damage or irritation of periwound skin.

Tissue damage related to chemical trauma

Chemical trauma may be caused by leakage or incontinence of body fluids, such as urine, feces, and exudate, or chemicals applied to the skin, such as lotions, iodine, soap, organic solvents, acids, and adhesives. Reactions to irritant contact dermatitis may vary widely from an itching rash similar to allergic contact dermatitis to cracks and fissures in the skin, especially on the hands, or denudement of skin, often in the perineal area. The skin reaction may be rapid and extremely painful. Treatment includes:

- Identifying irritant and eliminating contact with skin.
- Gentle cleansing of skin to remove irritant but avoid further skin irritation.
- Use of skin sealants or skin barriers as indicated to protect the skin and allow healing.
- Use of appropriate skin care products and containment devices.
- Monitoring of dressings and periwound condition daily.

Mechanical trauma

Mechanical trauma may result in stripping of the epidermis and sometimes the dermis of the skin or lacerations. Mechanical trauma may occur from tape removal or blunt trauma, such as colliding with furniture. Skin tears are categorized with the Payne-Martin Classification System:

1. Skin tear leaves avulsed skin adequate to cover wound. Tears may be linear or flap-type.
2. Skin tear with loss of partial thickness, involving either scant (<25% of epidermal flap over tear is lost) to moderate-large (> 25% of dermis in tear is lost).

3. Skin tear with complete loss of tissue, involving a partial-thickness wound with no epidermal flap.

Treatment includes:
- Recognizing fragile skin and treating carefully.
- Applying emollients, skin sealants, and skin barriers as indicated.
- Applying and removing tape appropriately.
- Avoiding adhesives when possible.
- Using hydrocolloids, SteriStrips, and transparent dressings to stabilize flaps.

Bacterial infections

Folliculitis and impetigo
Folliculitis is bacterial infection of the hair follicles, often on the face, resulting in pustules, erythema, and crusts that are painful and itchy. Recently, there has been an increase in cases of community-acquired methicillin-resistant *Staphylococcus aureus* folliculitis infections. Folliculitis may occur as a primary or secondary infection and may result from chronic nasal colonization of *MRSA*. Treatment includes:
- Antibacterial soaps.
- Topical or oral antibiotics.

Impetigo is a contagious itchy bacterial infection of the skin, commonly on the face or hands, causing clusters of blisters or sores, especially in children. Group A Streptococcus usually causes small blisters that crust over. Staphylococcus aureus usually causes larger blisters that may be bullous and cause lesions 2-8cm in size that persist for months. Treatment includes:
- Avoid itching
- Gently cleanse area with soap and water.
- Topical Bactroban® 3 times daily until healed.

SSSS
Staphylococcal scalded skin syndrome (SSSS) is a superficial partial-thickness infection of the skin caused by toxins produced by a localized *Staphylococcus aureus* infection, resulting in generalized erythema followed in 24-48 hours with blisters that rupture and peel off, leaving large areas of superficial necrosis and denuded skin, giving the skin a burned or "scalded" appearance. It is most common in neonates and children under 5 but can affect adults who are immunocompromised or in renal failure. Pain is usually mild unless the infection is very widespread. Treatment includes:
- IV antibiotics (such as flucloxacillin) are usually needed initially, followed by a course of oral antibiotics.
- Maintenance of fluids and electrolytes.
- Debridement of skin.

- Moisture-retentive dressings, such as foam dressings, sheet hydrogels, and alginates, avoiding adhesives.
- Excessive tissue loss may be treated the same as partial-thickness burns.

Erysipelas

Erysipelas is a superficial bacterial infection, primarily of the face or legs, involving the cutaneous lymphatic system and invading the skin in areas of trauma. Facial erysipelas is usually caused by group A *Streptococcus* following a nasopharyngeal infection. Infections on the legs are more often related to non-group A *Streptococcus.* The infection spreads rapidly with streaking and clearly demarcated erythema and cellulitis. Local lymph nodes become inflamed, sometimes resulting in lymphedema because of damage to lymph nodes. Erysipelas most commonly affects children and the elderly. Treatment includes:

- Bed rest with elevation of affected limb and warm saline packs to improve circulation.
- Oral antibiotic (usually penicillin G and penicillin VK). IV antibiotics may be indicated for severe cases.
- Hospitalization is recommended for severe cases or those who are very young, elderly, or immunocompromised.
- Analgesics to control pain.

Necrotizing fasciitis

Necrotizing fascitis is a rapidly spreading infection of the soft tissues involving extensive necrosis of the fascia and subcutaneous tissue as well as destruction of the vasculature with thrombosis. It most often occurs in the extremities after a minor infection. The most common organisms are group A β-hemolytic *Streptococci* but there may be polymicrobial infections or other causative agents. It may result from surgical procedures, including cardiac catheterization. The infection begins with pain, edema, fever, toxemia, and cellulitis that spreads rapidly, becoming increasingly cyanotic as tissue and perfusion is impaired. Bullae form and progress to necrosis and gangrene and sepsis within 3-5 days. Mortality rates are 25%. Treatment includes:

- Aggressive extensive surgical debridement of all non-viable tissue. Repeat surgical debridement may be necessary.
- Antibiotic therapy.
- Wound care as indicated by the extent of the wound with careful monitoring to determine if wound is deteriorating.
- IV immunoglobulin may be used.

Toxic shock syndrome

Toxic shock syndrome (TSS) is an acute severe life-threatening bacterial infection that causes a systemic infection with high fever, hypotension, myalgia, diarrhea and widespread erythematous rash that has the appearance of bad sunburn, with subsequent desquamation (peeling). The original causative agent was *Staphylococcus aureus* and infections were related to use of tampons, but the infection can occur with wounds or surgical sites where the bacteria can find entry. There are now 2 forms: *Staphylococcus aureus* (TSS) and *Streptococcal* toxic shock syndrome (STSS). *STSS* occurs secondary to an infection in the body, often an infected wound, causing severe hypotension, dyspnea, tachycardia, liver and kidney failure, and a splotchy rash that may peel. Treatment includes:

- Hospitalization for aggressive antibiotic therapy.
- Intravenous fluids to treat hypotension.
- Topical non-adhesive, non-occlusive dressings with absorbent materials as indicated.

Fungal infections

Candidiasis

Candidiasis, infection of the epidermis with *Candida* spp. (commonly referred to as "yeast" or "thrush"), causes a pustular erythematous papular rash that is commonly scaly, crusty, and macerated with a white cheese-like exudate. It may burn and is usually extremely pruritic and grows in warm moist areas of the skin, such as under breasts and abdominal folds and the perineal area. Antibiotic use, immunocompromised status, and diabetes mellitus may predispose people to fungal infections, so candidiasis must be differentiated from bacterial infections because antibiotic treatment will worsen the condition.

Treatment includes:

- Preventing humid moist conditions of skin.
- Controlling hyperglycemia.
- Burrows solutions soaks with air drying to relieve itching.
- Topical antifungal creams (clotrimazole, nystatin, fluconazole, and ketoconazole) twice daily.
- Topical antifungal powders for mild cases.
- Oral antifungal medications for severe cases.

Lymphedema

Medical management

Medical management of lymphedema *is* intended to reduce the protein accumulation in the tissues and restore lymphatic circulation, but treatment needs to begin before extensive fibrosis occurs. Diuretics do not help and the treatments must be carried out throughout lifetime in order to be successful:

- Hygiene: Skin must be kept clean and dry and inspected for open areas or signs of infection. Mild emollients may improve skin barrier.
- Antimicrobial or antifungal topical agents are used for infections. About 15-25% require long-term antibiotic prophylaxis.
- Limb elevation when possible and at night.
- Complex decongestive therapy with massage to improve lymphatic drainage.

- Static compression bandaging during the day, providing 40-60 mmHg pressure. May be removed at night if limb elevated.
- Dynamic compression (intermittent dynamic compression) may be used but can displace fluid or further damage lymphatics if not monitored carefully.
- Weight loss may be advised because obesity further compromises lymphatic circulation.

Patient management
Because management of lymphedema is a lifelong process, compliance on the part of the patient is critical to controlling lymphedema and preventing further deterioration and complications. The patient must take an active role:
- Avoid excessive heat, as in sun exposure, saunas, and hot tubs.
- Use electric razor instead of straight razor or chemicals for hair removal to prevent injury to skin.
- Prevent trauma to limb. Wear protective gloves and clothing to prevent trauma to affected limb. Avoid blood tests or blood pressure readings in an affected arm.
- Observe skin carefully for signs of cellulitis or infection and follow prescribed protocols for treatment.
- Maintain good hygiene.
- Wear closed-toe shoes if lower limb affected.
- Use sunscreen and bug repellent on affected limb.
- Avoid lifting and limit use of affected arm.

Venous dermatitis

Venous dermatitis appears on the ankles and lower legs and can cause severe itching and pain, and without treatment to control the dermatitis, it may deteriorate, causing ulcers to form, so treatment is needed to alleviate the symptoms:
- Topical antihistamines to decrease itching and prevent excoriation from scratching. Low dose topical steroids should be used only for short periods (2 weeks) to reduce inflammation and itching only because of danger of increasing ulceration.
- Compression therapy, usually with compression stockings, to affected legs to improve overall venous return.
- Leg elevation when sitting to avoid dependency.
- Topical antibiotics, such as bacitracin, as indicated to reduce danger of infection. Oral antibiotics as indicated for systemic infection.
- Hypoallergenic emollients (without perfume), such as petrolatum jelly, to improve the skin's barrier function is a preventive measure that should be used when the acute inflammation has subsided.

Edema

Chronic venous insufficiency results in edema of the lower extremities, causing both discomfort and increased risk of ulcers. Treatment includes:

- Leg elevation when sitting to avoid dependency. Therapy may include lying down and elevating affected limb above the heart for 1-2 hours two times daily and during the night. This is important for all patients with CVI, but especially for those unable to comply with compression therapy.
- Compression therapy, the type dependent upon the degree of edema.
- Surgical intervention is indicated if more conservative treatment are unsuccessful in managing insufficiency:
    - Ligation and stripping removes a vein or section of a vein that is damaged or has damaged valves. An incision below the vein allows an endoscope to be threaded into the vein to grasp and remove (strip) it. The vein is tied (ligated). Sometimes only ligation of a faulty valve is done and the vein is left in place.
    - Deep vein reconstruction may be considered if other approaches fail.
- Physical therapy is important because effective calf muscle pumping requires ankle mobility with dorsiflexion over 90°. Some patients may benefit from gait training and exercises to improve the range of motion and strength of the ankle. Calf muscle exercises may include isotonic exercises. Patients need to alternate sitting and standing with walking on a regular schedule throughout the day.
- Control of weight often improves circulation and reduces edema, as obesity may be the primary cause of the circulatory impairment. Patients may need education and referral to bariatric treatment center.
- Medications can't correct venous insufficiency but some can help to control symptoms:
    - Pentoxifylline (Trental®) enhances blood flow in capillaries.
    - Horse chestnut seed extract (HCSE) results in reduced pain and edema. It is widely used in Europe and has been studied in the United States. One problem is that it can cause low blood glucose levels in children and those with diabetes.

Measures to maximize perfusion

Lifestyle changes

The patient with arterial insufficiency must make lifestyle changes in order to avoid serious complications and/or amputation of the affected limb:

- Maintain adequate hydration to decrease blood viscosity, but avoid caffeine, which is vasoconstrictive.
- Pain control in order to prevent further vasoconstriction.
- Stop smoking as nicotine has vasoconstrictive properties.
- Begin a graduated walking program to improve tissue oxygenation, decrease pain, and increase activity tolerance.

- Avoid cold and constrictive clothing to avoid vasoconstriction.
- Do careful skin inspection and skin care, drying skin, using emollients and lamb's wool or foam between toes.
- Wear properly fitted, closed-toe shoes and avoid going barefoot.
- Have professional foot and nail care.
- Wear warm socks during cold weather, but avoid hot water bottles, heating pads, or hot bathing temperatures.
- Avoid the use of antiseptics or chemicals except as prescribed.
- Report even small injuries or changes in skin promptly.

Pharmacologic measures

The primary focus of pharmacologic measures to maximize perfusion is to reduce the risk of thromboses:

- Antiplatelet agents such as aspirin, Ticlid®, and Plavix® interfere with the function of the plasma membrane, interfering with clotting. These agents are ineffective to treat clots but prevent clot formation.
- Vasodilators may divert blood from ischemic areas, but some may be indicated, such as Pietal®, which dilates arteries and decreases clotting, and is used for control of intermittent claudication.
- Antilipemic, such as Zocor® and Questran®, slow progression of atherosclerosis.
- Hemorrheologics, such as Trental®, reduce fibrinogen, reducing blood viscosity and rigidity of erythrocytes; however, clinical studies show limited benefit. It may be used for intermittent claudication.
- Analgesics may be necessary to improve quality of life. Opioids may be needed in some cases.
- Thrombolytics may be injected into a blocked artery under angiography to dissolve clots.
- Anticoagulants, such as Coumadin® and Lovenox®, prevent blood clots from forming.

Preventing infection

Procedures for wound care should prevent infection of the wound and should prevent spread of infection to others. A clean "no-touch" method for dressing changes and wound care is currently recommended. Clean gloves (rather than sterile) are used, but dressings, gauze, swabs, or solutions that directly contact the open area of the wound should be sterile. Any container, such as a syringe or squeeze bottle, used to irrigate the wound should be sterile as well. Wound should be kept clean and debrided. Antimicrobials should be used as indicated and wound cultures done. Standard precautions should be used with handwashing both before and after treatment of wound, even with glove use, and before contact with other parts of the body. If any wound irrigation is done that involves fluid under pressure, staff should wear personal protective equipment (gloves, gown, mask, eye shield) to protect them and other patients from contamination with infective material.

Important terms

Amorphous — Lacking a defined form

Angiogenesis — Formation of new blood vessels and capillaries.

Autolysis — Destruction of body cells through the actions of macrophages and/or enzymes.

Cellulitis — Inflammation of tissue, usually with edema and pronounced erythema.

Debridement — Removal of necrotic tissue, devitalized tissue, or foreign material from a wound through surgical, mechanical, or other means.

Eschar — Dark brown or black leathery necrotic tissue.

Epithelization — Formation of healed tissue from epidermal cells over granulation.

Granulation — Bright pink or red granular appearing new tissue formed from capillary
beds.

Maceration — Softening and irritation caused by contact with liquid.

Necrosis — Dead tissue.

Occlusive — Impermeable to air or liquids.

Permeable — Allowing the passage of air and liquids.

Semi-permeable — Allowing the passage of water vapor and air (small ions or molecules).

Slough — Soft viscous yellow layer of necrotic tissue which covers and adheres to the wound.

Education and Training

Assessment of patient's educational needs

Assessment of the learner is critical in determining the educational needs for wound care or any type of self-care:

- Sensory abilities: Deficits in hearing or vision may impair a patient's ability to carry out wound care or to understand instructions. Provisions may be needed to compensate for deficits.
- Fine and gross motor skills: Patients must be able to manipulate supplies and carry out procedures necessary for wound care, and this may require some degree of mobility.
- Learning needs: The case manager should identify the learner, choose the correct setting, collect data to determine needs, and prioritize needs, involving other members of the team.
- Learning readiness: The 4 types of readiness to be assessed include physical (including sensory and motor skills), emotional, experiential, and knowledge.
- Learning style: The patient's learning style should be assessed to determine the type of delivery that would be most effective to meet the patient's educational needs.

Educating healthcare workers

Educating healthcare workers regarding wound care includes:

- Preventive measures: This includes frequency and methods of turning and positioning patients to prevent pressure sores and promote healing and information about skin appearance and impaired circulation. All healthcare workers should be cognizant of infection control practices and aware of the importance of hand washing.
- Complications: This includes tunneling, fistulae, abscesses, and local and systemic infections.
- Wound assessment: This includes not only noting complications but also measuring and monitoring for changes in size and condition.
- Use of assessment tools: Workers should be trained in the use of the Braden Scale and PUSH scale or any appropriate scale used by the facility to assess risk of pressure sores and to monitor the progress of wounds.
- Medicare/Medicaid requirements: As appropriate, healthcare workers (such as professional nursing staff) should be aware of coding issues related to reimbursement for wound care.

Controlling risk factors

Teaching patients and caregivers about risk factors and prevention strategies is an important part of wound management:

- Limited mobility: Referral for physical or occupational therapy may be indicated. If patients are unable to change position, caregivers must be taught proper skin care and positioning.
- Diabetes: Proper glucose monitoring and control is critical. Patients should avoid going barefoot and should inspect feet daily.
- Impaired circulation: Exercises may be indicated. Proper positioning to increase circulation should be stressed. Restrictive socks or clothing should be avoided.
- Cognitive impairment: Caregiver should be advised of all necessary treatments and may need to institute safety measures and assist patient with hygiene.
- Malnutrition: Diet should be planned and explained and supplements provided. Meals-on-wheels or assistance for food preparation and eating may be necessary.
- Fecal and urinary contamination: Medical and dietary instructions should be given to control incontinence, including scheduled voiding. Skin barriers may be needed as well assistance with hygiene and adult diapers.

Discharge plan for patient requiring wound care

The discharge planning should ideally begin when the patient is admitted to an inpatient facility so that the patient's needs can be carefully assessed. The important components of a discharge plan for a patient that requires wound care include:

- Education regarding wound appearance and signs of complications: Patient/family members should be able to recognize signs of impaired healing or infection.
- Education in infection control: Handwashing, clean technique for wound care.
- Written/Illustrated step-by-step instructions for wound care: Any procedures that the patient/family need to carry out should be fully outlined so they can be referred to during wound care.
- Bathing instructions: Any limitations (such as avoiding soaking the wound in a tub) should be noted.
- Referral to social worker (if necessary): Needs will depend on patient's age, living situation, and general condition.
- Referral to home health agency (if necessary): Nursing care, home health aide, physical therapy, occupational therapy.
- Follow-up plans: Physicians, return visits, return diagnostic tests.

Legal, Ethics, and Policy

Liability risks

Liability risks include the medical attention giver/patient association, communication, and educated approval or permission, clinical proficiency, self-assessment for experts regarding the necessity of keeping up-to-date records, consultation and medical appointment recommendations, guidelines, standard actions, modus operandi, and management of other people.

Malpractice

Malpractice includes an expert acting wrongly, inability to do a skill (that should reasonably be expected), disloyalty during work or in a position of trust, acting against the law to the detriment of the patient, or acting in an immoral way to the detriment of the patient. Malpractice also includes alleged professional not giving medical attention and not acting with conscientiousness or taking preventative measures that someone else in the identical industry would give to the patient to stop someone from becoming harmed. Negligence is not doing what a sensible practitioner would do in a case where a patient is harmed due to this inaction.

Signs of abuse

Regular screening for domestic violence in a healthcare setting is a helpful and inoffensive method of identifying victims. Watch for injuries that do not seem to match the story given. Overbearing or overprotective partners who answer for or dominate your interview with the patient, frequent nonspecific complaints such as headache, stomach, neck and back pain, insecurity, stammering or avoidance in giving responses to simple questions, intestinal complaints, and sexually transmitted disease. In the abused adolescent female tobacco, alcohol and drug use, decreased school attendance, isolation, and bulimia are more common.

Photographing wounds

While photographing wounds can provide a good visual record, the photographs should always be an addition to documented descriptions rather than a substitution, and there are ethical considerations. The patient must give informed consent for photography and should have a clear understanding of the purpose of the photography as well as who will have access to the photographs, how they can be accessed, and under which circumstances. As with all personal health information (PHI), safeguards should be in place to protect the patient's right to privacy and confidentiality. Institutions or healthcare practitioners who utilize photography of wounds should have clear guidelines that specify the conditions for photography, the equipment, criteria for who can take the photographs, and the type of patient identification that will be included. Provision must also be made for patients to obtain copies of any photographs upon request. Because state laws vary, the nurse should review any state requirements related to photography to ensure compliance.

Stark Law

The Stark Law was a provision of the Omnibus Budget Reconciliation Act (OBRA) (1989) under which the Medicare program banned self-referrals for laboratory services (Stark I). Self-referral occurs when a physician refers a patient for services at a facility in which the physician has a financial interest. Revision of OBRA (1993) expanded the law to cover other health services and applied the law to both Medicare and Medicaid (Stark II). Under the final rules (2009), per-click fee payments related to space or equipment leases are prohibited, so a physician cannot profit from referring a patient to a facility to which the physician leases space or equipment although some time-block leasing agreements are accepted. The new rulings also prohibit profiting from percentage-based leasing of space and equipment. Under the Affordable Care Act, while Stark allows physicians to refer patients for imaging services within a group practice, patients must be notified that they can choose to have the imaging done in other facilities.

Informed consent

Patients or guardians must provide informed consent for all treatment the patient receives. This includes a thorough explanation of all procedures and treatment and associated risks. Patients/guardians should be apprised of all options and allowed input on the type of treatments. Patients/guardians should be apprised of all reasonable risks and any complications that might be life threatening or increase morbidity. The American Medical Association has established guidelines for informed consent:
- Explanation of diagnosis.
- Nature and reason for treatment or procedure.
- Risks and benefits.
- Alternative options (regardless of cost or insurance coverage).
- Risks and benefits of alternative options.
- Risks and benefits of not having a treatment or procedure.
- Providing informed consent is a requirement of all states.

Advance directives

An advance directive is a way that a patient can communicate to his/her family and physician what kind of medical intervention he/she desires. Advance directives are legal documents and the specific laws regarding them vary by state. A patient must be competent in order to make an advance directive. A living will is a type of advance directive. It generally describes what type of intervention a patient desires in the face of terminal illness. A "Do Not Resuscitate" or DNR order is another type of advance directive. A DNR order must be written in the patient's chart by the attending physician in order to be valid. All discussions with the patient and the family should be clearly documented in the chart. In the absence of a written DNR order, call a full Code Blue and proceed with resuscitation.

HIPAA privacy directive

Privacy directives manage how patient's Protected Health Information (PHI) is utilized and given out for times when the data might reveal who the patient is. HIPAA controlled PHI for people who work in the health profession, health plans and health care clearing houses. The aim is to give tough Federal shields for the right to privacy and keep the best medical attention possible. All data is protected. Under this rule, there is a covered entity including the people who do the medical attention that communicate data electronically (as in billing, claims, or paying issues), health plans, and health care clearinghouses. Utilization and giving out of the protected information has to be done to the patient when he asks for it, to HHS, or to check up on or find out if the rule is being complied to. It is allowed for the patient, treatment, payment and healthcare operations (TPO), with the chance to concur or not, public policy, "incident to", restricted information set, and with permission.

Patient's/family's rights and responsibilities

Empowering patients and families to act as their own advocates requires they have a clear understanding of their rights and responsibilities. These should be given (in print form) and/or presented (audio/video) to patients and families on admission or as soon as possible:
- Rights should include competent, non-discriminatory medical care that respects privacy and allows participation in decisions about care and the right to refuse care. They should have clear understandable explanations of treatments, options, and conditions, including outcomes. They should be apprised of transfers, changes in care plan, and advance directives. They should have access to medical records information about charges.
- Responsibilities should including providing honest and thorough information about health issues and medical history. They should ask for clarification if they don't understand information that is provided to them, and they should follow the plan of care that is outlined or explain why that is not possible. They should treat staff and other patients with respect.

Patients' (families') rights in relation to what they should expect from a healthcare organization are outlined in both standards of the Joint Commission and National Committee for Quality Assurance. Rights include:

- Respect for patient, including personal dignity and psychosocial, spiritual, and cultural considerations.
- Response to needs related to access and pain control.
- Ability to make decisions about care, including informed consent, advance directives, and end of life care.
- Procedure for registering complaints or grievances.
- Protection of confidentiality and privacy.
- Freedom from abuse or neglect.
- Protection during research and information related to ethical issues of research.
- Appraisal of outcomes, including unexpected outcomes.
- Information about organization, services, and practitioners.
- Appeal procedures for decisions regarding benefits and quality of care.
- Organizational code of ethical behavior.
- Procedures for donating and procuring organs/tissue.

Culturally competent health care

Cultural sensitivity is an important attribute for APRNs and other clinicians to possess; ignorance of other cultural beliefs can lead to alienation of the patient, which will obviously compromise the therapeutic relationship and the overall healing process. An APRN who is culturally sensitive, moreover, does not make assumptions about cultures based on broad generalizations and stereotypes. Although there may be characteristics that seem to apply to a specific culture as a whole, it is important for the APRN to remember that each person has his or her own beliefs and attitudes, regardless of cultural differences. An APRN who practices culturally competent health care is attentive and intuitive, and is able to recognize how the patient is feeling based on the patient's behavior, even if the behavior is unexpected.

Communication and cultural awareness

Communication is a vital part of the APRN-patient relationship; of course, as any APRN knows, establishing open communication can be difficult with any patient, even if the patient and the APRN share similar beliefs and belong to the same cultural group. When the APRN is treating a patient of another culture, especially if there is a language barrier, communication can be frustrating for both the patient and the APRN. The APRN must exercise patience when communicating, and should explore different methods of communication if one does not seem to be working. It is important that the APRN always keep in mind that the goal is to provide the best treatment possible for the patient, and that education of the patient is paramount to recovery.

Effects of cultural diversity on assessment

Issues of cultural diversity must be considered during assessment. Individuals vary considerably in their attitudes, so assuming that all members of an ethnic or cultural group share the same values is never valid. The individual must be assessed as well as the group. It's important to take time to observe family dynamics and language barriers, arranging for translators if necessary to ensure that there is adequate communication. In patriarchal cultures, such as the Mexican culture, the eldest male may speak for the patient. In some Muslim cultures, females will resist care by males. Acknowledging biological differences, such as skin color, is important for assessing skin because wounds and bruising may have a different appearance. The attitudes and beliefs of the patient in relation to wound care must be understood, accepted, and treated with respect. In some cases, the use of healers or cultural traditions must be incorporated into a plan of care.

Documenting wounds

Legal requirements for documenting wounds are often quite general, requiring that documentation be "timely and accurate" without specifying exactly what that entails. However, CMS reimbursement is predicated on documented information, so correct documentation has, in effect, become a legal requirement. Considerations include:
- Coding for supplies utilized for wound care must be correct.
- Wounds must be coded properly as traumatic or nontraumatic.
- Debridement must be specified as excisional or nonexcisional.
- Laboratory and imaging reports and nutritional assessments that support wound care must be in the patient's health record.
- Wound size and stage must be documented in order to determine the patient's acuity level.
- Skin condition must be documented on admission, including any wounds that are present or lack of wounds.

General rules for charting should also be followed, including recording the date and time of all entries, using accurate measurements, providing factual objective information, and using only approved abbreviations in order to prevent errors.

Practice Test

Practice Questions

1. Which of the following extends from a wound under normal tissue and connects two structures, such as the wound and an organ?
    a. Undermining
    b. Fistula
    c. Tunneling
    d. Abscess

2. A patient has a wound on the right hip with tunneling and fistulae. Which of the following is *MOST* indicative of an abscess formation?
    a. Increased purulent discharge
    b. Increased wound pain
    c. Increased erythema and swelling at wound perimeter
    d. Erythematous, painful, swollen area 3 cm from wound perimeter

3. Which of the following laboratory tests is the most effective to monitor acute changes in nutritional status?
    a. Total protein
    b. Albumin
    c. Prealbumin
    d. Transferrin

4. On the eighth day of wound care, granulation tissue is evident about the wound perimeter, and the wound is beginning to contract. The wound is in which of the following phases of healing?
    a. Proliferation
    b. Inflammation
    c. Hemostasis
    d. Maturation

5. Which of the following is the correct procedure for applying Eutectic Mixture of Local Anesthetics (EMLA Cream) to a wound prior to debridement?
    a. Apply a thin layer (1/8 inch thick) to the wound for 15 minutes, leaving the wound open
    b. Apply a thick layer (1/4 inch thick) to the wound, extending 1/2 inch past the wound onto surrounding tissue, and cover with plastic wrap for 20 to 60 minutes
    c. Apply a thick layer (1/4 inch thick) to the wound surface only and cover with plastic wrap for 15 minutes
    d. Apply a thin layer (1/8 inch thick) to the wound surface only and cover with a loose dry dressing for 20 to 60 minutes

6. When doing a routine dressing change for a healing decubitus ulcer on the right hip, which is the most appropriate cleaning solution?
    a. Povidone-iodine solution
    b. Hydrogen peroxide
    c. Alcohol
    d. Normal saline

7. Which of the following wound irrigation devices will provide approximately 8 psi in irrigant pressure to the wound surface?
    a. 35-mL syringe with 19-gauge Angiocath
    b. 250-mL squeeze bottle
    c. Bulb syringe
    d. 6-mL syringe with 19-gauge Angiocath

8. Which of the following is the most important criterion when assessing a patient's level of wound pain?
    a. Patient's behavior
    b. Type of wound
    c. Patient's report of pain
    d. Patient's facial expression

9. Which of the following is likely to have the *MOST* negative effect on wound healing for a 65-year-old woman?
    a. Hypoalbuminemia
    b. BMI of 20.2
    c. BMI of 28
    d. Vegan diet

10 Which of the following is the most definitive method for obtaining a wound specimen for culture and sensitivities?
    a. Tissue biopsy
    b. Sterile swab of wound
    c. Needle biopsy
    d. Sterile swab of discharge

11. A patient with an infected abdominal wound is taking a number of drugs. Which of the following is most likely to impair healing?
    a. Phenytoin
    b. Corticosteroid
    c. Prostaglandin
    d. Estrogen

12. A burn extending through the dermis with obvious blistering would be classified as:
    a. First degree
    b. Second degree
    c. Third degree
    d. Full thickness

13. Which of the following results from smoking cigarettes?
    a. Vasodilation
    b. Vasoconstriction
    c. Increased oxygen transport
    d. Increased oxygen tension

14. When calculating the ankle-brachial index (ABI), if the ankle systolic pressure is 90 and the brachial systolic pressure is 120, what is the ABI?
    a. 1.33
    b. 13.3
    c. 7.5
    d. 0.75

15. Using transcutaneous oxygen pressure measurement (TCPO$_2$), which of the following values indicates that oxygenation is adequate for healing?
    a. 18 mm Hg
    b. 20 mm Hg
    c. 30 mm Hg
    d. 42 mm Hg

16. The method of closure that involves leaving the wound open and allowing it to close naturally through granulation and epithelialization is healing by:
    a. Primary or first intention
    b. Secondary or second intention
    c. Tertiary or third intention
    d. Quaternary prevention

17. A patient's laboratory results show increased serum sodium and serum osmolality. The most likely cause is:
    a. Infection
    b. Overhydration
    c. Dehydration
    d. Malnutrition

18. Autolytic debridement is most effective for:
    a. Chronic wounds
    b. Large burns
    c. Small wounds without infection
    d. Necrotic wounds

19. Enzymatic debridement requires application of enzymes:
    a. 1 to 2 times daily
    b. 3 to 4 times daily
    c. 1 to 2 times weekly
    d. 3 to 4 times weekly

20. Which of the following indicates that sharp instrument debridement must be discontinued?
    a. Purulent discharge occurs
    b. Black eschar is removed
    c. Pain and bleeding occur
    d. Patient complains of fatigue

21. A patient has second and third degree burns on 30% of the body and is in severe pain. Which method of debridement is most indicated?
    a. Autolytic debridement
    b. Enzymatic debridement
    c. Sharp instrument debridement
    d. Surgical debridement

22. Which method of mechanical debridement may cause damage to granulation tissue and is generally contraindicated?
    a. Wet to dry dressings
    b. Whirlpool bath
    c. Irrigation under pressure
    d. Ultrasound treatment

23 Which of the following topical antimicrobials is most appropriate to treat nasal colonization of *Staphylococcus aureus* in a patient with an open wound?
    a. Cadexomer iodine
    b. Metronidazole
    c. Mupirocin (Bactroban®)
    d. Silver sulfadiazine

24. Which of the following is a contraindication to negative pressure wound therapy?
    a. Chronic Stage IV pressure ulcer
    b. Wound malignancy
    c. Unresponsive arterial ulcer
    d. Dehiscent surgical wound

25. Which of the following is the primary goal in referring a patient for multidisciplinary consultation?
    a. Prevention of complications
    b. Treatment of complications
    c. Education
    d. Identification of outcomes

26. Becaplermin (Regranex®) gel, a growth factor, is indicated for which type of wound?
    a. Venous stasis ulcer
    b. Pressure ulcer
    c. Sutured/stapled wound
    d. Diabetic ulcer

27. Which of the following types of dressing is indicated for treatment of a full-thickness infected wound with large amount of exudate?
    a. Alginate
    b. Hydrocolloid
    c. Hydrogel
    d. Semipermeable film

28. What hyperbaric oxygen therapy (HBOT) treatment regimen is usually recommended for chronic wounds and lower extremity diabetic ulcers?
    a. Compression at 2 ATA 3 times 60 minutes daily for 48 hours
    b. Compression at 2 to 2.4 ATA for 90 minutes daily for at least 30 treatments
    c. Compression at 3 ATA for 2 to 4 hour periods 3 to 4 times daily
    d. Compression at 2 to 2.5 ATA for 60 to 90 minutes 2 times daily for 2 to 3 days and then decreasing frequency over 4 to 6 days

29. Which NPUAP stage is a pressure ulcer characterized by deep full-thickness ulceration that exposes subcutaneous tissue with possible presence of slough, tunneling, and undermining, but without visibility of underlying muscle, tendon, or bone?
    a. Stage I
    b. Stage II
    c. Stage III
    d. Stage IV

30. What is the most common cause of shear?
    a. "Sheet burn"
    b. Elevating the head of the bed >30°
    c. Lifting the patient with a pull sheet
    d. Turning the patient side to side

31. What is the minimal thickness of a support surface for a chair?
    a. One inch
    b. Two inches
    c. Three inches
    d. Four inches

32. When turning and repositioning patients, what is the preferred position for the patient to reduce pressure?
    a. Prone
    b. Supine
    c. 30° lateral
    d. 90° side lying

33. On the Braden scale for predicting risk of developing pressure scores, a patient scores 2 (1 to 4 or 1 to 3 scale) on each of 6 parameters (total score 12). What is the patient's risk of developing a pressure sore?
    a. Very minimal risk
    b. Breakpoint for risk
    c. High risk
    d. Extremely high risk (worst score)

34. Which type of overlay support surface is best for moisture control?
    a. Rubber
    b. Plastic
    c. Gel
    d. Foam

35. Which of the following characteristics indicates venous insufficiency?
    a. Pain ranges from intermittent to severe constant.
    b. Pulses are absent or weak.
    c. Brownish discoloration is evident about ankles and anterior tibial area
    d. Rubor occurs on dependency and pallor on foot elevation.

36. Which of the following is a typical example of a peripheral ulcer caused by arterial insufficiency?
    a. Deep, circular, necrotic ulcer on toe tips
    b. Irregular ulcer on medial malleolus
    c. Round ulcer on anterior tibial area
    d. Irregular ulcer on lateral malleolus

37. When assessing for capillary refill, arterial occlusion is indicated with refill time of:
    a. 15 seconds
    b. <2 seconds
    c. >20 seconds
    d. >2 to 3 seconds

38. A pulse graded as 1 on a 0 to 4 scale of intensity could be described as:
    a. Strong and bounding
    b. Weak, difficult to palpate
    c. Absent
    d. Normal, as expected

39. Which of the following off-loading measures is usually the **MOST** effective for treatment of neuropathic ulcers?
    a. Total contact cast
    b. Removable cast walkers
    c. Wheelchairs
    d. Half-shoes

40. Which of the following is characteristic of Charcot's arthropathy (Charcot's foot)?
    a. Severe pain and inflammation
    b. High arch and hypersensitivity
    c. Muscle spasms, increased pain, and inflammation
    d. Weak muscles, reduced sensation, inflammation, and collapsed arch

41. Which of the following is necessary to manage peripheral lymphedema of the legs?
    a. Daily diuretics
    b. Static compression bandaging
    c. Off-loading
    d. Bed rest

42. Which measurement must be used to evaluate the safety of static compression therapy to manage edema?
    a. Capillary refill time
    b. Venous refill time
    c. Ankle-brachial index
    d. Blood pressure

43. Which of the following pharmacological measures is used to maximize perfusion with intermittent claudication?
    a. Antiplatelet agents, such as Plavix®
    b. Vasodilators, such as cilostazol (Pletal®)
    c. Thrombolytics
    d. Anticoagulants, such as warfarin (Coumadin®)

44. Which of the following may be a subtle indication of infection with arterial insufficiency?
    a. Fever and chills:
    b. Decrease in necrotic area
    c. Decreased pain or edema
    d. Fluctuance of periwound tissue

45. A patient with venous insufficiency requires compression therapy and has Unna's boot applied but must be on bed rest for four weeks. Which action is correct?
    a. Continue Unna's boot therapy during bed rest, but change 2 times weekly
    b. Continue Unna's boot therapy, but keep leg elevated
    c. Discontinue Unna's boot therapy during the bed rest period
    d. Continue Unna's boot therapy, but change only every 2 weeks

46. When doing the nylon monofilament test, how many test sites should be used?
    a. 2
    b. 4
    c. 8
    d. 10

47. The *NEXT* step in wound care for a traumatic wound, such as a dog bite, after stabilizing the patient's condition and stopping bleeding is
    a. Administer antibiotics
    b. Administer tetanus toxoid/immune globulin as indicated
    c. Flush wound with copious amounts of normal saline under pressure
    d. Scrub wound with povidone-iodine

48. A patient with pemphigus vulgaris has generalized lesions with ulcerations and crusting, causing the patient's skin to adhere to the bed sheets. How can the patient manage this?
    a. Apply talcum powder liberally to the sheets
    b. Set an alarm to turn frequently during the night
    c. Place a piece of soft plastic over the sheets
    d. Use an alternating pressure mattress

49. What is the most effective treatment for a fungating neoplastic wound of the breast that is oozing blood from eroded vasculature?
    a. Charcoal dressing
    b. Hemostatic dressing and cauterization with silver nitrate
    c. Cleansing with ionic solution
    d. Surgical debridement

50. One of the primary treatments for contact dermatitis with an itching, blistering rash is
    a. Nonadherent dressings
    b. Topical corticosteroid
    c. Antibiotics
    d. Cleansing with povidone-iodine

Answers and Explanations

1. B: A fistula extends under normal tissue away from the wound and connects two structures, such as the wound and an organ or the wound and the skin. Undermining occurs when damaged tissue lies underneath intact skin about the wound perimeter. Tunneling is damaged tissue extending from the wound under normal tissue, but not opening to the skin or other structures. An abscess is a collection of purulent material in a localized area, often occurring with a fistula.

2. D: Abscesses often form in conjunction with fistulae. Typical indications include erythema, pain, and swelling above the localized area of the abscess. If the abscess is deep within the tissue or within an internal organ, however, obvious signs of abscess formation may not be evident, and symptoms may be less specific, including general malaise, abdominal pain, chills, fever, lethargy, diarrhea, and anorexia. Additional symptoms may be specific to the site of the abscess, for example a perirenal abscess may cause flank pain.

3. C: Prealbumin is most commonly monitored for acute changes in nutritional status because it has a half-life of only 2 to 3 days. Prealbumin decreases quickly when nutrition is inadequate and rises quickly in response to increased protein intake. Protein intake must be adequate to maintain normal levels of prealbumin.
- Normal value: 16 to 40 mg/dL.
- Mild deficiency: 10 to 15mg/dL
- Moderate deficiency: 5 to 9 mg/dL.
- Severe deficiency: <5 mg/dL.

Total protein levels and transferrin levels may be influenced by many factors, so they are not reliable measures of nutritional status. Albumin has a half-life of 18 to 20 days, so it is more sensitive to long-term protein deficiencies than to short-term deficiencies.

4. A: Proliferation (days 5 to 20) is characterized by granulation tissue starting to form at wound perimeter, contracting the wound, and epithelialization, resulting in scar formation. Hemostasis (within minutes) occurs as platelets seal off the vessels and the clotting mechanism begins. Inflammation (days 1 to days 4 to 6) is characterized by erythema and edema as phagocytosis removes debris. During maturation or remodeling (days 21 plus), scar tissue continues to form until the scar has about 80% of original tissue strength, and the wound closes; the underlying tissue continues to remodel for up to 18 months.

5. B: Eutectic Mixture of Local Anesthetics (EMLA Cream) is applied thickly (1/4 inch) to both the surface of the wound and surrounding tissue, extending about 1/2 inch past the wound. After application, the wound must be covered with plastic wrap for 20 to 60 minutes to numb the tissue. EMLA cream is effective for about an

hour after the wrapping is removed. EMLA can interact with a number of different medications, such as antiarrhythmics, anticonvulsants, and acetaminophen, so medications should be carefully reviewed prior to administration.

6. D: Normal saline is the most appropriate wound-cleansing solution. Antiseptic solutions should be avoided, as they may damage granulation tissue and retard healing, because they interfere with fibroblast cells necessary for healing of the wound, cause increased pain, and do not significantly reduce overall bacterial load. In heavily-contaminated or necrotic wounds, topical antiseptic solutions, such as dilute povidone-iodine or hydrogen peroxide, may be used for a short period of time to reduce surface bacteria and foul odor.

7. A: A 35-mL syringe with 19-gauge needle provides irrigation pressure at about 8 psi. A squeeze bottle (250 mL) provides about 4.5 psi, but a bulb syringe usually only ≤2 psi. Both syringe/catheter and needle size affect irrigant pressure. Pressures <4 psi do not provide adequate wound cleansing, but pressures >15 psi can result in wound trauma.
- 6 mL/19 gauge = 30 psi
- 12 mL/19 gauge = 20 psi
- 12 mL/22 gauge = 13 psi
- 35mL/21 gauge = 6 psi
- 35mL/25 gauge = 4 psi

8. C: Perceptions and expressions of pain vary widely from one individual to another, so the most important criterion for evaluating pain is the patient's own report of pain. Cultural differences have a role in how people express pain, with some cultures typically appearing more stoic than others. Using a 1 to 10 pain scale is an effective tool for people who are cognitively alert. If people are not able to report their pain level, then observation of behavior and facial expressions may give clues to their need for pain medication.

9. A: Hypoalbuminemia is likely to have the most negative effect on wound healing. Hypoalbuminemia is an indication of protein malnutrition (kwashiorkor) and may cause delayed wound healing because of inadequate nutrition. A BMI of 20.2 is within normal range (18.5 to 24.9) and indicates normal weight. A person with a BMI of 29 is overweight, but not obese. Both being underweight (BMI <18.5) and obese (BMI ≥30) can interfere with the body's ability to heal. BMI alone is not adequate to assess nutritional status or healing ability and vegan diets can provide adequate nutrition.

10. A: The most definitive method of obtaining a wound specimen for culture and sensitivities is with a tissue biopsy. A needle biopsy can also provide an adequate sample in many cases. Swabbing a wound with a sterile applicator often does not provide an adequate sample, because this method obtains material only from the wound surface, which may include both pathogenic agents from the wound and

contamination from skin bacteria. The tissue itself must be cultured, not just the discharge.

11. B: Corticosteroids may impair wound healing by interfering with vascular proliferation and epithelialization. The anti-inflammatory effect may interfere with the inflammatory phase of healing by decreasing migration of macrophages and polymorphonuclear leukocytes to the wound, interfering with angiogenesis, and increasing susceptibility to wound infection. Other drugs that may impair healing include vasoconstrictors, NSAIDs, aspirin, colchicine, immunosuppressant's, DMARDS (antirheumatoid arthritis drugs), and anticoagulants. Some drugs appear to promote wound healing, including phenytoin, prostaglandin, and estrogen.

12. B: A burn extending through the dermis with obvious blistering would be classified as a second-degree burn. A first-degree burn is superficial and involves only the epidermis. First and second-degree burns, like other wounds, may also be classified as partial-thickness injuries, because the vessels and glands necessary for healing remain intact. A third-degree burn, also classified as a full-thickness injury, extends through the dermis and into the underlying subcutaneous tissue and may extend through vessels, nerves, muscles and even to the bone.

13. B: The nicotine in cigarettes is a powerful vasoconstrictor and interferes with oxygen transport. The carbon monoxide from smoking displaces oxygen on hemoglobin, decreasing the level of oxygen in the blood. Vasoconstriction reduces delivery of nutrients needed for healing. Peripheral blood flow can be reduced by 50% for up to 60 minutes after smoking a cigarette, and oxygen tension may be reduced for 120 minutes. Additionally, nicotine increases the heart rate and blood pressure, so the heart requires more oxygen to function adequately, while receiving less.

14. D: The ankle-brachial index (ABI) examination evaluates peripheral arterial disease of the lower extremities. The ankle and brachial systolic pressures are obtained, and then the ankle systolic pressure is divided by the brachial systolic pressure to obtain the ABI. If the ankle systolic pressure is 90 and the brachial systolic pressure is 120: 90 divided by 120 = 0.75. Normal value is 1 to 1.1 with lower values indicating decreasing perfusion. A value of 0.75 indicates severe disease and ischemia.

15. D: Transcutaneous oxygen pressure measurement (TCPO$_2$) is a noninvasive test that measures dermal oxygen, to show the effectiveness of oxygen in the skin and tissues. A value of >40 mm Hg indicates adequate oxygenation for healing. Values of 20 to 40 mm Hg are equivocal findings, and values < 20 mm Hg indicate marked ischemia, affecting healing. Two or three different sites on the lower extremities should be tested to give a more accurate demonstration of oxygenation. TCPO$_2$ is often used to determine if oxygen transport is sufficient for hyperbaric therapy.

16. B: Secondary healing (healing by second intention) involves leaving the wound open and allowing it to close through granulation and epithelialization. Primary healing (healing by first intention) involves surgically closing a wound by suturing, flaps, or split or full-thickness grafts to completely cover the wound. Tertiary healing (healing by third intention) is also sometimes called delayed primary closure because it involves first debriding the wound and allowing it to begin healing while open and then later closing the wound through suturing or grafts. Quaternary prevention includes activities to prevent iatrogenic disorders/effects.

17. C: Increased serum sodium and serum osmolality indicate dehydration. Serum sodium measures the sodium level in the blood.
- Normal values: 135 to 150 mEq/L
- Dehydration: >150 mEq/L

Serum osmolality measures the concentration of ions, such as sodium, chloride, potassium, glucose, and urea in the blood. Levels increase with dehydration, which stimulates the antidiuretic hormone, resulting in increased water reabsorption and more concentrated urine in an effort to compensate.
- Normal levels: 285 to 295 mill-osmoles per kilogram/ H_2O
- Dehydration: >295 mOsm/kg/ H_2O

18. C: Autolytic debridement is effective for small wounds without infection, but it is slower than other types of debridement. Autolytic debridement requires an occlusive or semiocclusive dressing to create a warm moist wound environment. Any moisture-retentive dressing, such as hydrocolloids, alginate, and hydrogels, and transparent film, can promote some degree of autolytic debridement, but because of drainage and odor, surrounding tissue must be protected with some type of skin barrier to prevent tissue maceration.

19. A: Enzymatic (chemical) debridement requires application of enzymes 1 to 2 times daily and is most effective for a wound with necrosis and eschar, which must be crosshatched if it is dry. Enzymes include the following:
- Collagenase, applied 1 time daily. Wound pH must remain at 6 to 8 or the enzyme deactivates. Deactivated by Burrows solutions, hexachlorophene, and heavy metals.
- Papain/urea combinations, applied 1 to 2 times daily. Wound pH must remain at 3 to 12. Deactivated by hydrogen peroxide and heavy metals.

20. C: Pain and bleeding indicate that viable tissue is being débrided, so debridement must be discontinued. Only necrotic tissue/eschar should be removed by sharp debridement, removing small layers at a time to prevent injury to viable tissue. Purulent discharge often occurs with an infected wound. While patient fatigue is a concern, positioning the patient for comfort, explaining the procedure, and reassuring the patient may help the patient tolerate continuing the procedure until the wound is adequately débrided.

21. D: Surgical debridement is most commonly used when very large amounts of tissue must be débrided, such as with extensive burns or when there is immediate debridement is needed in order to effectively treat a serious wound infection. General anesthesia allows extensive debridement to be done without the patient suffering associated pain and trauma, although postoperative pain is common. One advantage is that most debridement can be done in one procedure. Lasers may also be used for surgical debridement, with pulsed lasers posing less risk to adjacent tissue than continuous lasers.

22. A: In the past, wet-to-dry gauze dressing were frequently used for wound care; but wet-to-dry dressings have little use in current wound care unless the wound is very small, because the gauze adheres to the wound and can disrupt granulation or epithelization. While a whirlpool bath may effectively cleanse debris from a wound, concerns about cross infection have resulted in less frequent use of the whirlpool. Ultrasound may effectively débride wounds. Irrigating a wound with pressurized solution can be effective if the pressure remains in the optimal range, usually 8 to 12 psi.

23. C: Mupirocin is effective against Gram-positive organisms, such as *Staphylococcus aureus* and MRSA, and is used for treating nasal colonization to decrease risk of wound infection. Cadexomer iodine is effective against a wide range of bacteria (staph, MRSA, strep, and pseudomonas), viruses, and fungi and is placed in the wound where beads of iodine swell in contact with exudate, releasing the iodine into the wound. Metronidazole is effective against bacterial infections, such as MRSA: Silver sulfadiazine is often used to treat burns and is effective against Gram-positive organisms, including Staph, MRSA, Strep, and Pseudomonas.

24. B: Contraindications to negative pressure wound therapy include wound malignancy, untreated osteomyelitis, exposed blood vessels or organs, and nonenteric, unexplored fistulas. Negative pressure therapy uses subatmospheric (negative) pressure with a suction unit and a semi occlusion vapor-permeable dressing. The suction reduces periwound and interstitial edema, decompressing vessels, improving circulation, stimulating production of new cells, increasing the rate of granulation and reepithelialization and decreasing colonization of bacteria NPWT is used for a variety of difficult-to-heal wounds, especially those that show less than 30% healing in 4 weeks of postdebridement treatment or those with excessive exudate.

25. A: The primary goal in referring a patient for multidisciplinary consultation is to prevent complications. A multidisciplinary team is composed of experts in a number of different fields, collaborating to address the complex problems associated with wound care and underlying pathology. Instead of the serial approach to problem solving involved in the traditional model of care, where referrals are made in response to problems that arise with little communication among specialists, the multidisciplinary approach attempts to identify potential problems and institute

preventive measures at the onset, with all members communicating and sharing information.

26. D: Becaplermin (Regranex®) gel is indicated for treatment of peripheral diabetic ulcers extending into subcutaneous tissue or deeper with adequate perfusion. Application follows debridement and usually about 3 weeks offloading if healing is not adequate. Becaplermin is a growth factor derived from human platelets. It is not approved for use with pressure ulcers and stasis ulcers and should not be used with closed (sutured/stapled) wounds. Becaplermin is associated with increased risk of developing malignancy and increased risk of death from existing malignancy.

27. A: Alginates are effective for infected full-thickness wounds with undermining, tunneling, and large amounts of exudate. They are made from brown seaweed and absorb exudate, forming a hydrophilic gel that conforms to the shape of the wound. Hydrocolloids are effective for clean wounds with granulation and minimal to moderate exudate, but they increase the risk of anaerobic infection and hypergranulation. Hydrogels are effective for partial- or full-thickness wounds that are dry or have a small amount of exudate. Hydrogels can be used with necrotic and infected wounds. Semipermeable film is effective over intravenous sites or dry, shallow, partial-thickness wounds.

28. B: The usual hyperbaric oxygen therapy (HBOT) for chronic wounds and lower extremity diabetic ulcers is compression at 2 to 2.4 ATA for 90 minutes daily, with at least 30 treatments. Oxygen toxicity may occur with treatment over 90 minutes. Hyperbaric oxygen therapy (HBOT) is treatment in a high-pressure chamber while breathing 100% oxygen, which increases available oxygen to tissues by 10 to 20 times, improving perfusion. HBOT results in
- Hyperoxygenation of blood and tissue
- Vasoconstriction, reducing capillary leakage
- Angiogenesis, because of increased fibroblasts and collagen
- Increased effectiveness of antibiotics needing active transport across cell walls (fluoroquinolone, amphotericin B, aminoglycosides)

29. C: This is a Stage III ulcer. NPUAP stages include
- Suspected deep tissue injury: purple/reddish discoloration and boggy, mushy, or firm tissue
- Stage I: skin intact with localized nonblanching reddened area, often over bony prominences
- Stage II: abrasion, blister, or slightly depressed area with red/pink wound bed, partial-thickness skin loss, but no slough
- Stage III: deep, full-thickness ulceration that exposes subcutaneous tissue with possible presence of slough, tunneling and undermining without visibility of underlying muscle, tendon, or bone
- Stage IV: deep, full-thickness ulceration with extensive damage, necrosis of tissue extending to muscle, bone, tendons, or joints

- Unstageable: cannot be staged before debridement because of the extent of slough/eschar

30. B: The most common cause of shear is elevation of the bed >30°. Shear occurs when the skin stays in place and the underlying tissue in the deep fascia over the bony prominences stretches and slides, damaging tissue and vessels, which become thrombosed, often resulting in undermining and deep ulceration. Friction against the sheets holds the skin in place while the body slides down the bed, causing pressure and damage in the sacrococcygeal area. The head of the bed should be maintained <30° except for the brief periods when the patient is lifted with a pull sheet or lifting device and turned, at least every 2 hours.

31. A: Support surface material should provide at least one inch of support under areas to be protected when in use to prevent "bottoming out." (Check by placing a hand palm up under the overlay, below the pressure point.). Static support surfaces are appropriate for patients who can change position without increasing pressure to an ulcer. Those needing assistance to move require dynamic support surfaces. Dynamic support surfaces are also needed when static pressure devices provide less than an inch of support.

32. C: The 30° lateral position is better than the 90° side-lying or supine positions because it prevents pressure over bony prominences. Prone (face down) is not comfortable for most patients and requires careful positioning. Devices such as pillows or foam should be used to correctly position patients so that bony prominences are protected and not in direct contact with each other. Patients should not be positioned on ulcers. Goals for repositioning and a turning schedule of at least every 2 hours should be established for each individual and documented.

33. C: A Braden score of 12 indicates high risk. The Braden scale rates 5 areas (sensory perception, moisture, activity, mobility, and usual nutrition pattern) with a 1 to 4 scale and one area (friction and shear) with a 1 to 3 scale. Lower scores correlate with increased risk. The scores for all six items are totaled, and a risk is assigned according to the number.
- 23 (best score): excellent prognosis with very minimal risk
- ≤16: breakpoint for risk of pressure ulcer (will vary somewhat for different populations)
- 12 to 14: high risk
- 6 (worst score): prognosis is very poor with strong likelihood of developing pressure ulcer

34. D: Foam overlays provide the best moisture control for preventing moisture damage to skin. Some materials, such as rubber, plastic, or gel, may increase perspiration and moisture, while some porous materials, including some types of foam, may reduce perspiration. Foam varies considerably in density and indentation load definition (ILD). ILD is the number of pounds of pressure needed to make an

- 115 -

indentation in a 4-inch foam of 25% of its thickness, using an indentation of 50 square inches. Foam can be closed-cell (resistant) or open cell (visco-elastic). Open-cell foam is temperature sensitive, helping it to mold to the body as it reaches the patient's body temperature.

35. C: Venous insufficiency is characterized by hemosiderin staining (brownish discoloration) about the ankles and anterior tibial area. Pain is usually aching and cramping, and peripheral pulses are present. Lipodermatosclerosis occurs in the lower leg area as the tissue becomes fibrotic from fibrin and protein (collagen) deposits, causing the skin to feel waxy and the tissue to harden, with narrowing of the tissue around the ankle compared to proximal tissue above. Venous (stasis) dermatitis is inflammation of the epidermis and dermis, resulting in scaly, erythematous, crusty, weepy, itchy skin, usually in the lower leg (ankle and tibia).

36. A: Arterial ulcers are characterized by painful, deep, circular, often necrotic ulcers on toe tips, toe webs, heels or other pressure areas, with little edema of extremity. Because circulation is impaired, peripheral pulses are weak or absent and skin is pale, shiny, and cool with loss of hair on toes and feet and little edema. Nails are thick, with ridges. Rubor occurs on dependency and pallor on foot elevation. Venous ulcers, by contrast, are typically superficial, irregular ulcers on the medial or lateral malleolus and sometimes on the anterior tibial area, with varying pain and moderate to severe edema of extremity.

37. D: Capillary refill time >2 to 3 seconds indicates arterial occlusion. To assess capillary refill, grasp the toenail bed between the thumb and index finger and apply pressure for several seconds to cause blanching. Release the nail and count the seconds until the nail regains normal color. Check both feet and more than one nail bed. Assess venous refill time with the patient lying supine for a few moments and then have the patient sit with the feet dependent. Observe the veins on the dorsum of the foot and count the seconds before normal filling. Venous occlusion is indicated with times >20 seconds.

38. B: A pulse graded 1 would be weak and difficult to palpate. Pulses should first be evaluated with the patient in a supine position and then again with the legs dependent, checking bilaterally and proximally to distally to determine if the intensity of pulse decreases distally. Pedal pulses should be examined at both the posterior tibialis and the dorsalis pedis. The pulse should be evaluated for rate, rhythm, and intensity, which is usually graded on a 0 to 4 scale.
- 0 – pulse absent
- 1 – weak, difficult to palpate
- 2 – normal, as expected
- 3 – full
- 4 – strong and bounding

39. A: Total contact casts (TCC) encase the lower extremity in a walking cast that equalizes pressure of the plantar surface. The casts may have windows over pressure ulcers to allow observation and treatment. TCC is more successful than other off-loading measures, possibly because people restrict activity more. Removable cast walkers allow patients to remove the casts, but studies show that people only use them 28% of the time, decreasing effectiveness. Wheelchairs allow dependency of using a limb but prevent pressure. Half shoes may have a high walking heel with the front of the foot elevated off of the ground.

40. D: Charcot's arthropathy results from neuropathy that weakens the muscles of the foot and reduces sensation. As muscles supporting the bones weaken, the bones become weak and fracture easily. Because of the lack of sensation, the patient may be unaware of the fracture and continue to walk, causing further deformity. It causes inflammation, swelling, and increased temperature in the foot, and but usually no pain. In time, the joint dislocation causes the arch to collapse. Treatment includes
- Compression bandages for 2 to 3 weeks
- Total contact or non–weight-bearing cast for up to 9 months
- Gradual weight-bearing after skin has resumed its normal temperature

41. B: Lymphedema is managed with static compression bandaging during the day, providing 40 to 60 mmHg pressure. Bandaging maybe removed at night if the limb is elevated. Dynamic compression may be used, but it can displace fluid or further damage lymphatics if not monitored carefully. Diuretics do not help. Lymphedema is a dysfunction of the lymphatic system, resulting in a debilitating, progressive disease. Proteins, lipids, and fluids accumulate in interstitial spaces, causing pronounced induration, edema, and fibrosis of tissues, resulting in distention and thick fibrotic skin with orange discoloration (peau d'orange). Scaly keratotic debris collects, and the skin develops cracks and leaks of lymphatic fluid.

42. C: Static compression is contraindicated if the ankle brachial index (ABI) is <0.5. Compression therapy serves as a preventive and therapeutic treatment to eliminate edema. It is contraindicated in those with heart failure or peripheral arterial disease, because it may further impair compromised arterial circulation.
- High level compression provides therapeutic compression at 30 to 40 mmHg at the ankle. Some may provide pressure at 40 to 50 mmHg. ABI should be >0.8.
- Low level compression provides modified pressure up to 23mmHg at the ankle. ABI must be >0.5 and <0.8. While this level is less than therapeutic, even low levels of pressure may provide some therapeutic benefit.

43. B: While vasodilators may divert blood from ischemic areas, some, such as cilostazol (Pletal®) or pentoxifylline (Trental®), may be indicated. Vasodilators dilate arteries and decrease clotting and are used for control of intermittent claudication. If medications do not relieve symptoms, surgical intervention, such as

bypass grafts, angioplasty, and even amputation (if ischemia is irreversible) may be necessary. Surgery is indicated with ABI <0.5 or >0.5 if the patient fails to respond to medication and lifestyle changes, or with intolerable, incapacitating pain.

44. D: Subtle indications of infection with arterial insufficiency include fluctuance (soft, wavelike texture) of periwound tissue on palpation, increased pain in the ischemic limb, or ulcer and/or increased edema, increased area of necrosis, and slight erythema about wound perimeter. Because of the lack of circulation, the normal signs of inflammation and infection may not be evident with arterial insufficiency, so observing for subtle signs of infection is critically important. Prompt identification and treatment is necessary to prevent cellulitis and/or osteomyelitis, which might necessitate amputation.

45. C: Unna's boot (ViscoPaste®) is a gauze wrap impregnated with zinc oxide, glycerin, or gelatin to provide a supporting compression "boot" to support the calf muscle pump during ambulation, so it is not suitable for nonambulatory patients and should be discontinued during the bed rest period. The bandage must be applied carefully, without tension. It may either be left open to dry or covered with an elastic or self-adherent wrap. The dressings are changed according to individual needs, determined by a decrease in edema, the amount of exudate, and hygiene, with dressing changes ranging from twice weekly to once every other week.

46. D: The nylon monofilament test is evaluated according to how many of 10 test sites the patient is able to detect, with <4 indicative of decreased sensation. To test, use this procedure:
- Ask the patient to indicate when the monofilament pressure is felt.
- Grasp a length of #10 monofilament in the instrument provided.
- Touch the monofilament against the bottom of the foot and then press the monofilament into the foot until the line buckles.
- Test the great, 3rd, and 5th toes.
- Test the left, medial, and right areas of the ball of the foot
- Test the right and left of the arch.
- Test the middle of the heel.

47. C: Traumatic injuries are usually contaminated, and once the patient is stable and the bleeding is controlled, the wound should be flushed with copious amounts of isotonic normal saline under pressure (8 to 12 psi), usually 100 to 200 mL of irrigant per inch of wound. Prophylactic antibiotics may be given for 3 to 7 days for superficial wounds and up to 14 days with evidence of infection. Tetanus toxoid or tetanus immune globulin may be necessary if vaccination is not current. Animal bites may also require rabies postexposure prophylaxis (PEP).

48. A: Applying talcum powder liberally to the sheets may help keep the patient's skin from sticking to them. Pemphigus vulgaris (PV), an autoimmune disorder causing blistering of both the skin and the mucus membranes (presenting symptom

in 50 to 70% of patients), creates burn-like wounds, which may heal slowly or not at all, often starting in the mouth and genital areas. Untreated, the disorder can lead to death. Blisters on skin rupture, causing ulcerations, and those in folds may develop hypergranulation and crusting. Treatment includes corticosteroids, immunosuppressive drugs, and plasmapheresis to remove antibodies.

49. B: The ulcers of fungating neoplastic wounds bleed as the vasculature erodes so hemostatic dressings (gel foam, alginates) and cauterization with silver nitrate may be necessary. Using nonadherent dressings or long-term dressing reduces trauma. Charcoal dressings control odor, and ionic cleansers or antiseptics may be used to cleanse the wound. A foam, alginate, or hydrofiber dressing or wound pouch is used to manage exudate. Skin sealants, barrier ointments, and hydrocolloid wafers to anchor tape protect periwound tissue.

50. B: With contact dermatitis, topical corticosteroid is used to control inflammation and itching. Skin should be gently cleansed with water or oatmeal bath and left open without dressings. Antibiotics are needed only if a secondary infection occurs. Caladryl® lotion may relieve itching, and antihistamines may reduce allergic response. Contact dermatitis is a localized response to contact with an allergen, resulting in a rash that may blister and itch. Common allergens include poison oak, poison ivy, latex, benzocaine, nickel, and preservatives, but people may react to a wide range of items, preparations, and products.

Secret Key #1 - Time is Your Greatest Enemy

Pace Yourself

Wear a watch. At the beginning of the test, check the time (or start a chronometer on your watch to count the minutes), and check the time after every few questions to make sure you are "on schedule."

If you are forced to speed up, do it efficiently. Usually one or more answer choices can be eliminated without too much difficulty. Above all, don't panic. Don't speed up and just begin guessing at random choices. By pacing yourself, and continually monitoring your progress against your watch, you will always know exactly how far ahead or behind you are with your available time. If you find that you are one minute behind on the test, don't skip one question without spending any time on it, just to catch back up. Take 15 fewer seconds on the next four questions, and after four questions you'll have caught back up. Once you catch back up, you can continue working each problem at your normal pace.

Furthermore, don't dwell on the problems that you were rushed on. If a problem was taking up too much time and you made a hurried guess, it must be difficult. The difficult questions are the ones you are most likely to miss anyway, so it isn't a big loss. It is better to end with more time than you need than to run out of time.

Lastly, sometimes it is beneficial to slow down if you are constantly getting ahead of time. You are always more likely to catch a careless mistake by working more slowly than quickly, and among very high-scoring test takers (those who are likely to have lots of time left over), careless errors affect the score more than mastery of material.

Secret Key #2 - Guessing is not Guesswork

You probably know that guessing is a good idea. Unlike other standardized tests, there is no penalty for getting a wrong answer. Even if you have no idea about a question, you still have a 20-25% chance of getting it right.

Most test takers do not understand the impact that proper guessing can have on their score. Unless you score extremely high, guessing will significantly contribute to your final score.

Monkeys Take the Test

What most test takers don't realize is that to insure that 20-25% chance, you have to guess randomly. If you put 20 monkeys in a room to take this test, assuming they answered once per question and behaved themselves, on average they would get 20-25% of the questions correct. Put 20 test takers in the room, and the average will be much lower among guessed questions. Why?
1. The test writers intentionally write deceptive answer choices that "look" right. A test taker has no idea about a question, so he picks the "best looking" answer, which is often wrong. The monkey has no idea what looks good and what doesn't, so it will consistently be right about 20-25% of the time.
2. Test takers will eliminate answer choices from the guessing pool based on a hunch or intuition. Simple but correct answers often get excluded, leaving a 0% chance of being correct. The monkey has no clue, and often gets lucky with the best choice.

This is why the process of elimination endorsed by most test courses is flawed and detrimental to your performance. Test takers don't guess; they make an ignorant stab in the dark that is usually worse than random.

$5 Challenge

Let me introduce one of the most valuable ideas of this course—the $5 challenge:

You only mark your "best guess" if you are willing to bet $5 on it.
You only eliminate choices from guessing if you are willing to bet $5 on it.

Why $5? Five dollars is an amount of money that is small yet not insignificant, and can really add up fast (20 questions could cost you $100). Likewise, each answer choice on one question of the test will have a small impact on your overall score, but it can really add up to a lot of points in the end.

The process of elimination IS valuable. The following shows your chance of guessing it right:

If you eliminate wrong answer choices until only this many remain:	Chance of getting it correct:
1	100%
2	50%
3	33%

However, if you accidentally eliminate the right answer or go on a hunch for an incorrect answer, your chances drop dramatically—to 0%. By guessing among all the answer choices, you are GUARANTEED to have a shot at the right answer.

That's why the $5 test is so valuable. If you give up the advantage and safety of a pure guess, it had better be worth the risk.

What we still haven't covered is how to be sure that whatever guess you make is truly random. Here's the easiest way:

Always pick the first answer choice among those remaining.

Such a technique means that you have decided, **before you see a single test question**, exactly how you are going to guess, and since the order of choices tells you nothing about which one is correct, this guessing technique is perfectly random.

This section is not meant to scare you away from making educated guesses or eliminating choices; you just need to define when a choice is worth eliminating. The $5 test, along with a pre-defined random guessing strategy, is the best way to make sure you reap all of the benefits of guessing.

Secret Key #3 - Practice Smarter, Not Harder

Many test takers delay the test preparation process because they dread the awful amounts of practice time they think necessary to succeed on the test. We have refined an effective method that will take you only a fraction of the time.

There are a number of "obstacles" in the path to success. Among these are answering questions, finishing in time, and mastering test-taking strategies. All must be executed on the day of the test at peak performance, or your score will suffer. The test is a mental marathon that has a large impact on your future.

Just like a marathon runner, it is important to work your way up to the full challenge. So first you just worry about questions, and then time, and finally strategy:

Success Strategy

1. Find a good source for practice tests.
2. If you are willing to make a larger time investment, consider using more than one study guide. Often the different approaches of multiple authors will help you "get" difficult concepts.
3. Take a practice test with no time constraints, with all study helps, "open book." Take your time with questions and focus on applying strategies.
4. Take a practice test with time constraints, with all guides, "open book."
5. Take a final practice test without open material and with time limits.

If you have time to take more practice tests, just repeat step 5. By gradually exposing yourself to the full rigors of the test environment, you will condition your mind to the stress of test day and maximize your success.

Secret Key #4 - Prepare, Don't Procrastinate

Let me state an obvious fact: if you take the test three times, you will probably get three different scores. This is due to the way you feel on test day, the level of preparedness you have, and the version of the test you see. Despite the test writers' claims to the contrary, some versions of the test WILL be easier for you than others.

Since your future depends so much on your score, you should maximize your chances of success. In order to maximize the likelihood of success, you've got to prepare in advance. This means taking practice tests and spending time learning the information and test taking strategies you will need to succeed.

Never go take the actual test as a "practice" test, expecting that you can just take it again if you need to. Take all the practice tests you can on your own, but when you go to take the official test, be prepared, be focused, and do your best the first time!

Secret Key #5 - Test Yourself

Everyone knows that time is money. There is no need to spend too much of your time or too little of your time preparing for the test. You should only spend as much of your precious time preparing as is necessary for you to get the score you need.

Once you have taken a practice test under real conditions of time constraints, then you will know if you are ready for the test or not.

If you have scored extremely high the first time that you take the practice test, then there is not much point in spending countless hours studying. You are already there.

Benchmark your abilities by retaking practice tests and seeing how much you have improved. Once you consistently score high enough to guarantee success, then you are ready.

If you have scored well below where you need, then knuckle down and begin studying in earnest. Check your improvement regularly through the use of practice tests under real conditions. Above all, don't worry, panic, or give up. The key is perseverance!

Then, when you go to take the test, remain confident and remember how well you did on the practice tests. If you can score high enough on a practice test, then you can do the same on the real thing.

General Strategies

The most important thing you can do is to ignore your fears and jump into the test immediately. Do not be overwhelmed by any strange-sounding terms. You have to jump into the test like jumping into a pool—all at once is the easiest way.

Make Predictions

As you read and understand the question, try to guess what the answer will be. Remember that several of the answer choices are wrong, and once you begin reading them, your mind will immediately become cluttered with answer choices designed to throw you off. Your mind is typically the most focused immediately after you have read the question and digested its contents. If you can, try to predict what the correct answer will be. You may be surprised at what you can predict.

Quickly scan the choices and see if your prediction is in the listed answer choices. If it is, then you can be quite confident that you have the right answer. It still won't hurt to check the other answer choices, but most of the time, you've got it!

Answer the Question

It may seem obvious to only pick answer choices that answer the question, but the test writers can create some excellent answer choices that are wrong. Don't pick an answer just because it sounds right, or you believe it to be true. It MUST answer the question. Once you've made your selection, always go back and check it against the question and make sure that you didn't misread the question and that the answer choice does answer the question posed.

Benchmark

After you read the first answer choice, decide if you think it sounds correct or not. If it doesn't, move on to the next answer choice. If it does, mentally mark that answer choice. This doesn't mean that you've definitely selected it as your answer choice, it just means that it's the best you've seen thus far. Go ahead and read the next choice. If the next choice is worse than the one you've already selected, keep going to the next answer choice. If the next choice is better than the choice you've already selected, mentally mark the new answer choice as your best guess.

The first answer choice that you select becomes your standard. Every other answer choice must be benchmarked against that standard. That choice is correct until proven otherwise by another answer choice beating it out. Once you've decided that no other answer choice seems as good, do one final check to ensure that your answer choice answers the question posed.

Valid Information

Don't discount any of the information provided in the question. Every piece of information may be necessary to determine the correct answer. None of the information in the question is there to throw you off (while the answer choices will certainly have information to throw you off). If two seemingly unrelated topics are discussed, don't ignore either. You can be confident there is a relationship, or it wouldn't be included in the question, and you are probably going to have to determine what is that relationship to find the answer.

Avoid "Fact Traps"

Don't get distracted by a choice that is factually true. Your search is for the answer that answers the question. Stay focused and don't fall for an answer that is true but irrelevant. Always go back to the question and make sure you're choosing an answer that actually answers the question and is not just a true statement. An answer can be factually correct, but it MUST answer the question asked. Additionally, two answers can both be seemingly correct, so be sure to read all of the answer choices, and make sure that you get the one that BEST answers the question.

Milk the Question

Some of the questions may throw you completely off. They might deal with a subject you have not been exposed to, or one that you haven't reviewed in years. While your lack of knowledge about the subject will be a hindrance, the question itself can give you many clues that will help you find the correct answer. Read the question carefully and look for clues. Watch particularly for adjectives and nouns describing difficult terms or words that you don't recognize. Regardless of whether you completely understand a word or not, replacing it with a synonym, either provided or one you more familiar with, may help you to understand what the questions are asking. Rather than wracking your mind about specific detailed information concerning a difficult term or word, try to use mental substitutes that are easier to understand.

The Trap of Familiarity

Don't just choose a word because you recognize it. On difficult questions, you may not recognize a number of words in the answer choices. The test writers don't put "make-believe" words on the test, so don't think that just because you only recognize all the words in one answer choice that that answer choice must be correct. If you only recognize words in one answer choice, then focus on that one. Is it correct? Try your best to determine if it is correct. If it is, that's great. If not, eliminate it. Each word and answer choice you eliminate increases your chances of getting the question correct, even if you then have to guess among the unfamiliar choices.

Eliminate Answers

Eliminate choices as soon as you realize they are wrong. But be careful! Make sure you consider all of the possible answer choices. Just because one appears right, doesn't mean that the next one won't be even better! The test writers will usually put more than one good answer choice for every question, so read all of them. Don't worry if you are stuck between two that seem right. By getting down to just two remaining possible choices, your odds are now 50/50. Rather than wasting too much time, play the odds. You are guessing, but guessing wisely because you've been able to knock out some of the answer choices that you know are wrong. If you are eliminating choices and realize that the last answer choice you are left with is also obviously wrong, don't panic. Start over and consider each choice again. There may easily be something that you missed the first time and will realize on the second pass.

Tough Questions

If you are stumped on a problem or it appears too hard or too difficult, don't waste time. Move on! Remember though, if you can quickly check for obviously incorrect answer choices, your chances of guessing correctly are greatly improved. Before you completely give up, at least try to knock out a couple of possible answers. Eliminate what you can and then guess at the remaining answer choices before moving on.

Brainstorm

If you get stuck on a difficult question, spend a few seconds quickly brainstorming. Run through the complete list of possible answer choices. Look at each choice and ask yourself, "Could this answer the question satisfactorily?" Go through each answer choice and consider it independently of the others. By systematically going through all possibilities, you may find something that you would otherwise overlook. Remember though that when you get stuck, it's important to try to keep moving.

Read Carefully

Understand the problem. Read the question and answer choices carefully. Don't miss the question because you misread the terms. You have plenty of time to read each question thoroughly and make sure you understand what is being asked. Yet a happy medium must be attained, so don't waste too much time. You must read carefully, but efficiently.

Face Value

When in doubt, use common sense. Always accept the situation in the problem at face value. Don't read too much into it. These problems will not require you to make huge leaps of logic. The test writers aren't trying to throw you off with a cheap trick. If you have to go beyond creativity and make a leap of logic in order to have an answer choice answer the question, then you should look at the other answer choices. Don't overcomplicate the problem by creating theoretical relationships or explanations that will warp time or space. These are normal problems rooted in reality. It's just that the applicable relationship or explanation may not be readily apparent and you have to figure things out. Use your common sense to interpret anything that isn't clear.

Prefixes

If you're having trouble with a word in the question or answer choices, try dissecting it. Take advantage of every clue that the word might include. Prefixes and suffixes can be a huge help. Usually they allow you to determine a basic meaning. Pre- means before, post- means after, pro - is positive, de- is negative. From these prefixes and suffixes, you can get an idea of the general meaning of the word and try to put it into context. Beware though of any traps. Just because con- is the opposite of pro-, doesn't necessarily mean congress is the opposite of progress!

Hedge Phrases

Watch out for critical hedge phrases, led off with words such as "likely," "may," "can," "sometimes," "often," "almost," "mostly," "usually," "generally," "rarely," and "sometimes." Question writers insert these hedge phrases to cover every possibility. Often an answer choice will be wrong simply because it leaves no room for exception. Unless the situation calls for them, avoid answer choices that have definitive words like "exactly," and "always."

Switchback Words

Stay alert for "switchbacks." These are the words and phrases frequently used to alert you to shifts in thought. The most common switchback word is "but." Others include "although," "however," "nevertheless," "on the other hand," "even though," "while," "in spite of," "despite," and "regardless of."

New Information

Correct answer choices will rarely have completely new information included. Answer choices typically are straightforward reflections of the material asked about and will directly relate to the question. If a new piece of information is included in an answer choice that doesn't even seem to relate to the topic being asked about, then that answer choice is likely incorrect. All of the information needed to answer the question is usually provided for you in the question. You should not have to make guesses that are unsupported or choose answer choices that require unknown information that cannot be reasoned from what is given.

Time Management

On technical questions, don't get lost on the technical terms. Don't spend too much time on any one question. If you don't know what a term means, then odds are you aren't going to get much further since you don't have a dictionary. You should be able to immediately recognize whether or not you know a term. If you don't, work with the other clues that you have—the other answer choices and terms provided—but don't waste too much time trying to figure out a difficult term that you don't know.

Contextual Clues

Look for contextual clues. An answer can be right but not the correct answer. The contextual clues will help you find the answer that is most right and is correct. Understand the context in which a phrase or statement is made. This will help you make important distinctions.

Don't Panic

Panicking will not answer any questions for you; therefore, it isn't helpful. When you first see the question, if your mind goes blank, take a deep breath. Force yourself to mechanically go through the steps of solving the problem using the strategies you've learned.

Pace Yourself

Don't get clock fever. It's easy to be overwhelmed when you're looking at a page full of questions, your mind is full of random thoughts and feeling confused, and the clock is ticking down faster than you would like. Calm down and maintain the pace that you have set for yourself. As long as you are on track by monitoring your pace, you are guaranteed to have enough time for yourself. When you get to the last few minutes of the test, it may seem like you won't have enough time left, but if you only have as many questions as you should have left at that point, then you're right on track!

Answer Selection

The best way to pick an answer choice is to eliminate all of those that are wrong, until only one is left and confirm that is the correct answer. Sometimes though, an answer choice may immediately look right. Be careful! Take a second to make sure that the other choices are not equally obvious. Don't make a hasty mistake. There are only two times that you should stop before checking other answers. First is when you are positive that the answer choice you have selected is correct. Second is when time is almost out and you have to make a quick guess!

Check Your Work

Since you will probably not know every term listed and the answer to every question, it is important that you get credit for the ones that you do know. Don't miss any questions through careless mistakes. If at all possible, try to take a second to look back over your answer selection and make sure you've selected the correct answer choice and haven't made a costly careless mistake (such as marking an answer choice that you didn't mean to mark). The time it takes for this quick double check should more than pay for itself in caught mistakes.

Beware of Directly Quoted Answers

Sometimes an answer choice will repeat word for word a portion of the question or reference section. However, beware of such exact duplication. It may be a trap! More than likely, the correct choice will paraphrase or summarize a point, rather than being exactly the same wording.

Slang

Scientific sounding answers are better than slang ones. An answer choice that begins "To compare the outcomes..." is much more likely to be correct than one that begins "Because some people insisted..."

Extreme Statements

Avoid wild answers that throw out highly controversial ideas that are proclaimed as established fact. An answer choice that states the "process should used in certain situations, if…" is much more likely to be correct than one that states the "process should be discontinued completely." The first is a calm rational statement and doesn't even make a definitive, uncompromising stance, using a hedge word "if" to provide wiggle room, whereas the second choice is a radical idea and far more extreme.

Answer Choice Families

When you have two or more answer choices that are direct opposites or parallels, one of them is usually the correct answer. For instance, if one answer choice states "x increases" and another answer choice states "x decreases" or "y increases," then those two or three answer choices are very similar in construction and fall into the same family of answer choices. A family of answer choices consists of two or three answer choices, very similar in construction, but often with directly opposite meanings. Usually the correct answer choice will be in that family of answer choices. The "odd man out" or answer choice that doesn't seem to fit the parallel construction of the other answer choices is more likely to be incorrect.

Special Report: How to Overcome Test Anxiety

The very nature of tests caters to some level of anxiety, nervousness, or tension, just as we feel for any important event that occurs in our lives. A little bit of anxiety or nervousness can be a good thing. It helps us with motivation, and makes achievement just that much sweeter. However, too much anxiety can be a problem, especially if it hinders our ability to function and perform.

"Test anxiety," is the term that refers to the emotional reactions that some test-takers experience when faced with a test or exam. Having a fear of testing and exams is based upon a rational fear, since the test-taker's performance can shape the course of an academic career. Nevertheless, experiencing excessive fear of examinations will only interfere with the test-taker's ability to perform and chance to be successful.

There are a large variety of causes that can contribute to the development and sensation of test anxiety. These include, but are not limited to, lack of preparation and worrying about issues surrounding the test.

Lack of Preparation

Lack of preparation can be identified by the following behaviors or situations:

Not scheduling enough time to study, and therefore cramming the night before the test or exam
Managing time poorly, to create the sensation that there is not enough time to do everything
Failing to organize the text information in advance, so that the study material consists of the entire text and not simply the pertinent information
Poor overall studying habits

Worrying, on the other hand, can be related to both the test taker, or many other factors around him/her that will be affected by the results of the test. These include worrying about:

Previous performances on similar exams, or exams in general
How friends and other students are achieving
The negative consequences that will result from a poor grade or failure

There are three primary elements to test anxiety. Physical components, which involve the same typical bodily reactions as those to acute anxiety (to be discussed below). Emotional factors have to do with fear or panic. Mental or cognitive issues concerning attention spans and memory abilities.

Physical Signals

There are many different symptoms of test anxiety, and these are not limited to mental and emotional strain. Frequently there are a range of physical signals that will let a test taker know that he/she is suffering from test anxiety. These bodily changes can include the following:

Perspiring
Sweaty palms
Wet, trembling hands
Nausea
Dry mouth
A knot in the stomach
Headache
Faintness
Muscle tension
Aching shoulders, back and neck
Rapid heart beat
Feeling too hot/cold

To recognize the sensation of test anxiety, a test-taker should monitor him/herself for the following sensations:

The physical distress symptoms as listed above
Emotional sensitivity, expressing emotional feelings such as the need to cry or laugh too much, or a sensation of anger or helplessness
A decreased ability to think, causing the test-taker to blank out or have racing thoughts that are hard to organize or control.

Though most students will feel some level of anxiety when faced with a test or exam, the majority can cope with that anxiety and maintain it at a manageable level. However, those who cannot are faced with a very real and very serious condition, which can and should be controlled for the immeasurable benefit of this sufferer.

Naturally, these sensations lead to negative results for the testing experience. The most common effects of test anxiety have to do with nervousness and mental blocking.

Nervousness

Nervousness can appear in several different levels:

The test-taker's difficulty, or even inability to read and understand the questions on the test

The difficulty or inability to organize thoughts to a coherent form

The difficulty or inability to recall key words and concepts relating to the testing questions (especially essays)

The receipt of poor grades on a test, though the test material was well known by the test taker

Conversely, a person may also experience mental blocking, which involves:

Blanking out on test questions

Only remembering the correct answers to the questions when the test has already finished.

Fortunately for test anxiety sufferers, beating these feelings, to a large degree, has to do with proper preparation. When a test taker has a feeling of preparedness, then anxiety will be dramatically lessened.

The first step to resolving anxiety issues is to distinguish which of the two types of anxiety are being suffered. If the anxiety is a direct result of a lack of preparation, this should be considered a normal reaction, and the anxiety level (as opposed to the test results) shouldn't be anything to worry about. However, if, when adequately prepared, the test-taker still panics, blanks out, or seems to overreact, this is not a fully rational reaction. While this can be considered normal too, there are many ways to combat and overcome these effects.

Remember that anxiety cannot be entirely eliminated, however, there are ways to minimize it, to make the anxiety easier to manage. Preparation is one of the best ways to minimize test anxiety. Therefore the following techniques are wise in order to best fight off any anxiety that may want to build.

To begin with, try to avoid cramming before a test, whenever it is possible. By trying to memorize an entire term's worth of information in one day, you'll be shocking your system, and not giving yourself a very good chance to absorb the information. This is an easy path to anxiety, so for those who suffer from test anxiety, cramming should not even be considered an option.

Instead of cramming, work throughout the semester to combine all of the material which is presented throughout the semester, and work on it gradually as the course goes by, making sure to master the main concepts first, leaving minor details for a week or so before the test.

To study for the upcoming exam, be sure to pose questions that may be on the examination, to gauge the ability to answer them by integrating the ideas from your texts, notes and lectures, as well as any supplementary readings.

If it is truly impossible to cover all of the information that was covered in that particular term, concentrate on the most important portions, that can be covered very well. Learn these concepts as best as possible, so that when the test comes, a goal can be made to use these concepts as presentations of your knowledge.

In addition to study habits, changes in attitude are critical to beating a struggle with test anxiety. In fact, an improvement of the perspective over the entire test-taking experience can actually help a test taker to enjoy studying and therefore improve the overall experience. Be certain not to overemphasize the significance of the grade - know that the result of the test is neither a reflection of self worth, nor is it a measure of intelligence; one grade will not predict a person's future success.

To improve an overall testing outlook, the following steps should be tried:

Keeping in mind that the most reasonable expectation for taking a test is to expect to try to demonstrate as much of what you know as you possibly can. Reminding ourselves that a test is only one test; this is not the only one, and there will be others.
The thought of thinking of oneself in an irrational, all-or-nothing term should be avoided at all costs.
A reward should be designated for after the test, so there's something to look forward to. Whether it be going to a movie, going out to eat, or simply visiting friends, schedule it in advance, and do it no matter what result is expected on the exam.

Test-takers should also keep in mind that the basics are some of the most important things, even beyond anti-anxiety techniques and studying. Never neglect the basic social, emotional and biological needs, in order to try to absorb information. In order to best achieve, these three factors must be held as just as important as the studying itself.

Study Steps

Remember the following important steps for studying:

Maintain healthy nutrition and exercise habits. Continue both your recreational activities and social pass times. These both contribute to your physical and emotional well being.
Be certain to get a good amount of sleep, especially the night before the test, because when you're overtired you are not able to perform to the best of your best ability.
Keep the studying pace to a moderate level by taking breaks when they are needed, and varying the work whenever possible, to keep the mind fresh instead of getting bored.
When enough studying has been done that all the material that can be learned has been learned, and the test taker is prepared for the test, stop studying and do

something relaxing such as listening to music, watching a movie, or taking a warm bubble bath.

There are also many other techniques to minimize the uneasiness or apprehension that is experienced along with test anxiety before, during, or even after the examination. In fact, there are a great deal of things that can be done to stop anxiety from interfering with lifestyle and performance. Again, remember that anxiety will not be eliminated entirely, and it shouldn't be. Otherwise that "up" feeling for exams would not exist, and most of us depend on that sensation to perform better than usual. However, this anxiety has to be at a level that is manageable.

Of course, as we have just discussed, being prepared for the exam is half the battle right away. Attending all classes, finding out what knowledge will be expected on the exam, and knowing the exam schedules are easy steps to lowering anxiety. Keeping up with work will remove the need to cram, and efficient study habits will eliminate wasted time. Studying should be done in an ideal location for concentration, so that it is simple to become interested in the material and give it complete attention. A method such as SQ3R (Survey, Question, Read, Recite, Review) is a wonderful key to follow to make sure that the study habits are as effective as possible, especially in the case of learning from a textbook. Flashcards are great techniques for memorization. Learning to take good notes will mean that notes will be full of useful information, so that less sifting will need to be done to seek out what is pertinent for studying. Reviewing notes after class and then again on occasion will keep the information fresh in the mind. From notes that have been taken summary sheets and outlines can be made for simpler reviewing.

A study group can also be a very motivational and helpful place to study, as there will be a sharing of ideas, all of the minds can work together, to make sure that everyone understands, and the studying will be made more interesting because it will be a social occasion.

Basically, though, as long as the test-taker remains organized and self confident, with efficient study habits, less time will need to be spent studying, and higher grades will be achieved.

To become self confident, there are many useful steps. The first of these is "self talk." It has been shown through extensive research, that self-talk for students who suffer from test anxiety, should be well monitored, in order to make sure that it contributes to self confidence as opposed to sinking the student. Frequently the self talk of test-anxious students is negative or self-defeating, thinking that everyone else is smarter and faster, that they always mess up, and that if they don't do well, they'll fail the entire course. It is important to decreasing anxiety that awareness is made of self talk. Try writing any negative self thoughts and then disputing them with a positive statement instead. Begin self-encouragement as though it was a friend speaking. Repeat positive statements to help reprogram the mind to believing in successes instead of failures.

Helpful Techniques

Other extremely helpful techniques include:

Self-visualization of doing well and reaching goals
While aiming for an "A" level of understanding, don't try to "overprotect" by setting your expectations lower. This will only convince the mind to stop studying in order to meet the lower expectations.
Don't make comparisons with the results or habits of other students. These are individual factors, and different things work for different people, causing different results.
Strive to become an expert in learning what works well, and what can be done in order to improve. Consider collecting this data in a journal.
Create rewards for after studying instead of doing things before studying that will only turn into avoidance behaviors.
Make a practice of relaxing - by using methods such as progressive relaxation, self-hypnosis, guided imagery, etc - in order to make relaxation an automatic sensation.
Work on creating a state of relaxed concentration so that concentrating will take on the focus of the mind, so that none will be wasted on worrying.
Take good care of the physical self by eating well and getting enough sleep.
Plan in time for exercise and stick to this plan.

Beyond these techniques, there are other methods to be used before, during and after the test that will help the test-taker perform well in addition to overcoming anxiety.

Before the exam comes the academic preparation. This involves establishing a study schedule and beginning at least one week before the actual date of the test. By doing this, the anxiety of not having enough time to study for the test will be automatically eliminated. Moreover, this will make the studying a much more effective experience, ensuring that the learning will be an easier process. This relieves much undue pressure on the test-taker.

Summary sheets, note cards, and flash cards with the main concepts and examples of these main concepts should be prepared in advance of the actual studying time. A topic should never be eliminated from this process. By omitting a topic because it isn't expected to be on the test is only setting up the test-taker for anxiety should it actually appear on the exam. Utilize the course syllabus for laying out the topics that should be studied. Carefully go over the notes that were made in class, paying special attention to any of the issues that the professor took special care to emphasize while lecturing in class. In the textbooks, use the chapter review, or if possible, the chapter tests, to begin your review.

It may even be possible to ask the instructor what information will be covered on the exam, or what the format of the exam will be (for example, multiple choice, essay, free form, true-false). Additionally, see if it is possible to find out how many questions will be on the test. If a review sheet or sample test has been offered by the professor, make good use of it, above anything else, for the preparation for the test. Another great resource for getting to know the examination is reviewing tests from previous semesters. Use these tests to review, and aim to achieve a 100% score on each of the possible topics. With a few exceptions, the goal that you set for yourself is the highest one that you will reach.

Take all of the questions that were assigned as homework, and rework them to any other possible course material. The more problems reworked, the more skill and confidence will form as a result. When forming the solution to a problem, write out each of the steps. Don't simply do head work. By doing as many steps on paper as possible, much clarification and therefore confidence will be formed. Do this with as many homework problems as possible, before checking the answers. By checking the answer after each problem, a reinforcement will exist, that will not be on the exam. Study situations should be as exam-like as possible, to prime the test-taker's system for the experience. By waiting to check the answers at the end, a psychological advantage will be formed, to decrease the stress factor.

Another fantastic reason for not cramming is the avoidance of confusion in concepts, especially when it comes to mathematics. 8-10 hours of study will become one hundred percent more effective if it is spread out over a week or at least several days, instead of doing it all in one sitting. Recognize that the human brain requires time in order to assimilate new material, so frequent breaks and a span of study time over several days will be much more beneficial.

Additionally, don't study right up until the point of the exam. Studying should stop a minimum of one hour before the exam begins. This allows the brain to rest and put things in their proper order. This will also provide the time to become as relaxed as possible when going into the examination room. The test-taker will also have time to eat well and eat sensibly. Know that the brain needs food as much as the rest of the body. With enough food and enough sleep, as well as a relaxed attitude, the body and the mind are primed for success.

Avoid any anxious classmates who are talking about the exam. These students only spread anxiety, and are not worth sharing the anxious sentimentalities.

Before the test also involves creating a positive attitude, so mental preparation should also be a point of concentration. There are many keys to creating a positive attitude. Should fears become rushing in, make a visualization of taking the exam, doing well, and seeing an A written on the paper. Write out a list of affirmations that will bring a feeling of confidence, such as "I am doing well in my English class," "I studied well and know my material," "I enjoy this class." Even if the affirmations aren't believed at first, it sends a positive message to the subconscious which will result in an alteration of the overall belief system, which is the system that creates reality.

If a sensation of panic begins, work with the fear and imagine the very worst! Work through the entire scenario of not passing the test, failing the entire course, and dropping out of school, followed by not getting a job, and pushing a shopping cart through the dark alley where you'll live. This will place things into perspective! Then, practice deep breathing and create a visualization of the opposite situation - achieving an "A" on the exam, passing the entire course, receiving the degree at a graduation ceremony.

On the day of the test, there are many things to be done to ensure the best results, as well as the most calm outlook. The following stages are suggested in order to maximize test-taking potential:

Begin the examination day with a moderate breakfast, and avoid any coffee or beverages with caffeine if the test taker is prone to jitters. Even people who are used to managing caffeine can feel jittery or light-headed when it is taken on a test day.
Attempt to do something that is relaxing before the examination begins. As last minute cramming clouds the mastering of overall concepts, it is better to use this time to create a calming outlook.
Be certain to arrive at the test location well in advance, in order to provide time to select a location that is away from doors, windows and other distractions, as well as giving enough time to relax before the test begins.
Keep away from anxiety generating classmates who will upset the sensation of stability and relaxation that is being attempted before the exam.
Should the waiting period before the exam begins cause anxiety, create a self-distraction by reading a light magazine or something else that is relaxing and simple.

During the exam itself, read the entire exam from beginning to end, and find out how much time should be allotted to each individual problem. Once writing the exam, should more time be taken for a problem, it should be abandoned, in order to begin another problem. If there is time at the end, the unfinished problem can always be returned to and completed.

Read the instructions very carefully - twice - so that unpleasant surprises won't follow during or after the exam has ended.

When writing the exam, pretend that the situation is actually simply the completion of homework within a library, or at home. This will assist in forming a relaxed atmosphere, and will allow the brain extra focus for the complex thinking function.

Begin the exam with all of the questions with which the most confidence is felt. This will build the confidence level regarding the entire exam and will begin a quality momentum. This will also create encouragement for trying the problems where uncertainty resides.

Going with the "gut instinct" is always the way to go when solving a problem. Second guessing should be avoided at all costs. Have confidence in the ability to do well.

For essay questions, create an outline in advance that will keep the mind organized and make certain that all of the points are remembered. For multiple choice, read every answer, even if the correct one has been spotted - a better one may exist.

Continue at a pace that is reasonable and not rushed, in order to be able to work carefully. Provide enough time to go over the answers at the end, to check for small errors that can be corrected.

Should a feeling of panic begin, breathe deeply, and think of the feeling of the body releasing sand through its pores. Visualize a calm, peaceful place, and include all of the sights, sounds and sensations of this image. Continue the deep breathing, and take a few minutes to continue this with closed eyes. When all is well again, return to the test.

If a "blanking" occurs for a certain question, skip it and move on to the next question. There will be time to return to the other question later. Get everything done that can be done, first, to guarantee all the grades that can be compiled, and to build all of the confidence possible. Then return to the weaker questions to build the marks from there.

Remember, one's own reality can be created, so as long as the belief is there, success will follow. And remember: anxiety can happen later, right now, there's an exam to be written!

After the examination is complete, whether there is a feeling for a good grade or a bad grade, don't dwell on the exam, and be certain to follow through on the reward that was promised...and enjoy it! Don't dwell on any mistakes that have been made, as there is nothing that can be done at this point anyway.

Additionally, don't begin to study for the next test right away. Do something relaxing for a while, and let the mind relax and prepare itself to begin absorbing information again.

From the results of the exam - both the grade and the entire experience, be certain to learn from what has gone on. Perfect studying habits and work some more on confidence in order to make the next examination experience even better than the last one.

Learn to avoid places where openings occurred for laziness, procrastination and day dreaming.

Use the time between this exam and the next one to better learn to relax, even learning to relax on cue, so that any anxiety can be controlled during the next exam. Learn how to relax the body. Slouch in your chair if that helps. Tighten and then relax all of the different muscle groups, one group at a time, beginning with the feet and then working all the way up to the neck and face. This will ultimately relax the muscles more than they were to begin with. Learn how to breathe deeply and comfortably, and focus on this breathing going in and out as a relaxing thought. With every exhale, repeat the word "relax."

As common as test anxiety is, it is very possible to overcome it. Make yourself one of the test-takers who overcome this frustrating hindrance.

Additional Bonus Material

Due to our efforts to try to keep this book to a manageable length, we've created a link that will give you access to all of your additional bonus material.

Please visit http://www.mometrix.com/bonus948/wcc to access the information.